BALDNESS, GRAYNESS—
Treatable or Nontreatable?

BALDNESS, GRAYNESS—
Treatable or Nontreatable?

by

Anthony J. Parrotto

WHITMORE PUBLISHING CO.
PITTSBURGH, PENNSYLVANIA 15222

All Rights Reserved
Copyright © 2005 by Anthony J. Parrotto
No part of this book may be reproduced or transmitted
in any form or by any means, electronic or mechanical,
including photocopying, recording, or by any information
storage and retrieval system without permission in
writing from the author.

ISBN # 87426-001-9
Printed in the United States of America

Second Printing

For information or to order additional books, please write:
Whitmore Publishing Co.
926 Liberty Avenue
Pittsburgh, Pennsylvania 15222
U.S.A.
Or visit our web site and online catalogue at www.whitmorebooks.com

Contents

	PAGE
INTRODUCTION	7

PART I

TRUTHS AND FALLACIES ABOUT HAIR AND SCALP PROBLEMS

1. Common Fallacies 13
2. Facts About Hair Care 17
3. Facts About Hair Products 22
4. Hair and Scalp Clinics 27
5. Medical Doctors and Hair and Scalp Problems 33

PART II

UNDERSTAND HAIR AND SCALP PROBLEMS; RECOGNIZE YOUR OWN TYPE

6. How Hair and Scalp Problems May Be Classified 37
7. Grayness 40
8. Baldness 45
9. Scaliness of the Scalp 56
10. Oiliness of the Scalp 61
11. Other Common Scalp Problems 64

PART III

HAIR, HEREDITY, AND AGING

12. The Hair and Scalp and Aging 71
13. Heredity and Hair 83
14. Are You Growing Old Before Your Time? ... 91
15. Baldness, Grayness, Dandruff—Treatable or Nontreatable? 98

Introduction

Take equal measures of fat from the bodies of a lion, a hippo, a crocodile, a snake, and a goat. Mix well and heat. Apply to the top of a barren scalp.

Believe it or not, this is part of history's first recorded medical prescription. It is Egyptian and dates back some 5000 years. Its purpose: to stimulate a sprouting of what mankind has been trying desperately either to produce or to destroy ever since — human hair.

The reason has remained much the same through centuries of superstition and scientific investigation. Hair makes a difference in our personal attractiveness. The presence or the absence of hair and its radiant good health or lifelessness affects us in many ways. It can reinforce or weaken our business contacts, strengthen or sabotage our inner confidence and poise, enhance or frustrate our natural desire to succeed socially.

Of course the presence or the absence of hair does not have so much influence on everyone. Many strong-willed personalities surge ahead in life with an admirable disregard for personal appearance. Most of us, however, are sensitive about the image we present to the world, even though we have been told time and again that "beauty is only skin deep."

That we are concerned in this respect is truer today than ever before. Modern communications — particularly television — have made us more aware of our personal appearance. In fact, Madison Avenue advertising men have spent a great deal of money creating the illusion of a youthful, vigorous, and healthy average American. Consequently, more than ever before, we appreciate and try to cultivate the physical assets that we possess.

This is particularly true of our hair. There is strong evidence that we lavish more time, worry, and money on it than on any other part of the human body. It is little wonder, therefore, that we usually submit to every nostrum that enjoys contemporary favor when we are faced with a hair problem — especially thinning and graying.

In efforts to remedy a hair condition we may, at one time or another, follow the suggestions to pluck, singe, or shave the hair, cut it close, expose it to plenty of sunlight, avoid wearing a hat, go on special diets, or submit to other "tried and true" theories. We may take time to brush the hair carefully 100 strokes a day and to follow a rigid massaging schedule. Our scalps may become a proving ground for widely promoted tonics, special shampoos, vibrators, and other promising contrivances. And finally we may turn for help to the self-promoted "hair specialists" of the ill-famed hair and scalp clinics.

While it is the exception rather than the rule to consult a medical doctor, it seems that somewhere along the line most of us get the word from the world of science that we are foolish for resorting to such nostrums, because generally little can be done for the more common hair and scalp problems. The implication we get is that hair is of little importance to our welfare anyhow and that we should not be so vain. This suggestion, however, is not in keeping with the illusion created by Madison Avenue and accepted by most Americans, and it is hardly a substitute for the more convincing propositions of the pseudoscientists.

And so the search goes on, not so much by the up-to-date scientists in this field, perhaps, but by the millions of concerned victims and many medical doctors, as well as by barbers and beauticians who make hair their life work. The search goes on for answers to questions that have baffled curious men and women for centuries.

Are baldness, grayness, and dandruff treatable or nontreatable? And, if they are treatable, how?

In efforts to answer these questions about the various types of these hair problems, many books and articles have been written. None has been successful, however, in reaching the masses with an acceptable explanation of dandruff and the most common type of baldness and grayness — a fact readily confirmed by the prevalence of confusion, superstition, and quackery that still prevails.

This book succeeds where the others have failed because it answers all the key questions about hair problems without raising new questions, and because it is written in plain, nontechnical language that can be understood by everyone.

When these problems are thoroughly dissected, it is found that there are logical explanations. When scientific papers, books and articles, and folklore are studied — when hair-care techniques and hair products and treatments are evaluated — when personal interviews with medical men, barbers, beauticians, and the man on the street are analyzed — when all these disconnected facts are synthesized properly, it is found that there are answers . . . startling answers.

The fact becomes clear that literally millions of people unknowingly are developing common baldness, common grayness, and other characteristics of aging before they should — that is, prematurely; and that millions are afflicted with dandruff needlessly without realizing its significance.

The chapters that follow spell out these answers in

three parts. When you come to appreciate the significance of these answers, you will realize why, in this age of moon rockets and wonder drugs, medical men, barbers, and beauticians continue to ramble on about common baldness, common grayness, and dandruff, allowing confusion and anxiety to prevail and superstition and quackery to flourish — all unnecessarily.

A. J. P.

PART I

Truths and Fallacies about Hair and Scalp Problems

CHAPTER 1

Common Fallacies

There is strong evidence that the average person's knowledge about his hair is a conglomeration of superstition, half truths, and outright fallacies. This chapter reveals some of the more common fallacies and misconceptions about hair and explains why they overshadow knowledge of the truth.

Outright Fallacies and Superstitions

Probably the most famous of the myths concerning hair is the story of Samson. Although most of us heard this story when we were young and impressionable, there are not many who would admit belief in the theory that long hair gives a person strength. Yet other equally ridiculous ideas about human hair are believed by a great many persons.

The belief that wearing a hat indoors causes baldness because it offends a celestial being is a case in point. Another belief that borders on the ridiculous is that the finger of God has touched the man with a bald spot in the center of the scalp and he is therefore destined to be a priest. That the list is virtually endless can be seen from the following additional examples: (1) men should shave off their beards in order to prevent nourishment from being diverted from the scalp; (2) if hair is wetted to make it lie down, it will rot; and (3) sleeping in short beds will cause baldness. Certainly these ideas are worthy of little more than a hearty laugh, but it is a sobering thought to realize that they have been believed by some people.

Misconceptions

Some of the theories concerning hair involve a more "scientific" leaning and therefore seem more plausible on the surface. Take, for example, the idea that singeing the hair ends is preferable to cutting them. The reason given is that a canal or tube exists in the center of the hair shaft and that cutting the hairs leaves the ends open, allowing the fluid to drain from them. This loss, in turn, is supposed to cause a loss of strength which retards hair growth. Singeing, on the other hand, prevents the loss of this fluid by welding the hair end into a closed point, so the theory goes. Actually, this theory has absolutely no foundation. Hair is a spiny growth similar to human nails or horses' hooves and contains no fluid of any kind.

Another theory which seems logical upon first examination holds that baldness is caused by the growth of the brain. The expanding brain tissue supposedly presses the blood vessels of the scalp, cutting down the flow of nourishment to the hair-growing apparatus. What makes the brain grow? Why, thinking, of course! And the more intensive the thinking, the greater is the growth of the brain, supposedly. Not only is there no evidence of the brain's growing in this respect, but there is also the fact of such renowned full-time thinkers as Vannevar Bush, Alfred Kinsey, and Albert Einstein, to mention just three, who enjoyed a full head of hair along with thousands of other intellectuals.

A series of experiments conducted by a prominent school of medicine recently disposed of another long-standing misconception — namely, that sunlight beneficially influences the growth of hair. This notion was probably based on the common knowledge that sunshine makes all kinds of plant life grow. Unfortunately, this truism does not hold true for human hair.

One of the most time-honored propositions says that the wearing of a hat causes baldness. It restricts the flow of blood to the hair roots, so goes the theory, while the top of the hat encloses the hair in a stifling, sunless prison. Except when a hat is so tight that it actually does cut off circulation of the blood in the scalp, there is no danger to the hair. In fact, scientific studies have shown that it is the individual who does not wear a hat who runs the greater risk! Wind and sun may cause the hair to become so dry and brittle that it breaks easily.

A final example of popular misconceptions is the belief that cutting or shaving the hair affects its rate of growth. Actually, experimental investigators have shown conclusively that cutting or shaving have no beneficial effect on the rate of hair growth. This misconception may have been nourished by what we might call an "optical illusion." When the hair is 6 or 8 inches long, we barely notice its growth, but after a crew cut we can observe its growth almost daily. Hence the conviction that shortened hair grows faster than long hair.

Conclusion

While it would be difficult to estimate accurately the number of persons who believe these fallacies and misconceptions, the fact remains that they have existed or do exist among peoples everywhere. The major reason for their existence has been lack of accurate knowledge in this area. And it is only logical to expect that fallacies and misconceptions (such as those mentioned in this chapter and others not yet imagined) will continue to exist and be accepted by many until ignorance and confusion are replaced by a proper understanding of the true nature of common hair and scalp problems.

CHAPTER 2

Facts About Hair Care

Because our hair makes such a difference in our personal appearance, most of us try to treat it with care. This chapter discusses and evaluates some of the common methods and techniques of hair care.

Brushing and Massaging

Besides helping to keep the hair well groomed, brushing and massaging aid in maintaining a healthy environment for normal hair growth. They stimulate circulation, sending blood coursing through the blood vessels which supply nourishment to scalp tissues. Suppleness of the hair and scalp is increased, and scales and dirt particles are loosened which otherwise could lead to infection. In addition, the natural oil of the scalp is spread up the hair shafts, giving them a new luster.

With regard to brushing, the hair should be brushed for several minutes morning and night; this should leave the scalp glowing pink, but not sore and irritated. The full length of the hair should be brushed to clean it and to distribute the natural oil. It is best to brush under the hair and upward, lifting the hair and the scalp to exercise the latter. Remember, though, that violent tugging is unnecessary and only results in broken hair.

In choosing between a brush with nylon bristles and one with natural bristles, keep in mind the following facts. Nylon is a shiny, smooth substance, which means that its bristles cannot easily remove dirt from the hair. Some nylon brushes have bristles cut off square at the end, and these can easily abrade the scalp or break and pull out hair. A natural bristle, on the other hand, has imbrications similar to those of human hair. This means that it is better suited to help distribute the natural oil of the scalp and to remove the dirt that accumulates in the hair daily. No matter which type bristle you choose, however, you should clean the brush regularly.

With regard to massaging, you should rub and knead the scalp with the pads of the fingers or the mound on the palm just below the thumb. Enough pressure should be exerted to move the scalp over the skull, and the movement itself should be a gentle, circular motion. Be sure that it is the scalp that moves and not the fingers; merely running the fingers roughly through the hair will not benefit the scalp and may cause unnecessary breakage of hair. The scalp should be massaged carefully for several minutes each day.

Although brushing and massaging do aid in maintaining a healthy environment for normal hair growth, three important facts should be kept in mind:

1. If the scalp is normal, hair will grow healthfully even without the aid of brushing and massaging.

2. When the hair-growing area beneath the surface of the scalp is not provided with the proper "nourishment," no amount of brushing or massaging can in itself create the necessary nourishment.

3. When degenerative changes beneath the surface of the scalp result in hair loss or grayness, neither brushing nor massaging can in themselves check or reverse these changes. The answer to these problems lies elsewhere.

Shampooing

Cleanliness is an important requirement for a healthy scalp and healthy hair. As a collector of dirt, dust, grease, and soot, the hair ranks near the top when compared with other parts of the human body. People who insist that the hair should be washed only three or four times a year would be shocked if this schedule were proposed for bathing any other part of the body.

While brushing and massaging do help keep both hair and scalp clean, shampooing is the only thorough method. The superiority of shampooing can be likened to the cleaning of a kitchen floor by washing it with soap and water as opposed to merely sweeping it with a broom.

Unlike the other commercial aspects of hair treatment, the producers of shampoos have created a number of thoroughly satisfactory products. Most shampoos on the market are entirely adequate for most scalps, whether they are a soap, a synthetic cleaning agent, or a detergent. It remains only for the individual to observe whether his hair is on the dry or oily side. If oily, a detergent shampoo is recommended because it has a slight drying quality. On the other hand, a dry scalp would benefit most from a shampoo containing oil.

The manner in which the hair should be shampooed is usually specified on the particular shampoo. In any case, the final rinse should be a thorough one to insure that the hair and scalp are completely free of any soap particles. Failure to rinse thoroughly may result in the hair's taking on a dull appearance. The hair should be dried soon after shampooing. Excessive friction and highly concentrated heat should be avoided, however.

The main purpose of shampooing, of course, is to keep the hair and scalp clean. How frequently this should be done will depend, to a large extent, on the degree of oiliness and other individual factors. For most people once a week is adequate. Those who are exposed to a great deal of dirt and grit, however, should wash their hair more frequently. Then again, some persons may be exposed to certain chemicals and materials that can directly or indirectly affect the hair and scalp, and, unless these offending substances are avoided, even daily shampooing will not be sufficient to overcome their adverse effects.

In addition to cleaning, shampooing helps to maintain a healthy environment for normal hair growth. Nevertheless, remember that (1) no amount of proper shampooing followed by careful drying can do any basic harm if the hair and scalp are in a healthy condition; (2) in cases of abnormal oiliness, dryness, and/or dandruff, no cure can be expected from frequent or infrequent shampooing. This is true of even specially "medicated" shampoos. The answer to these problems is not found in shampooing.

Hair Coloring and Permanent Waving

It is not the purpose of this book to describe the processes of hair coloring or permanent waving, but only to comment on their relationship to the health of the hair.

These practices are not harmful to the hair if administered skillfully and used with discretion. A woman has far more reason to insist on the skill of her beautician than a man of his barber. Cutting the hair merely shortens it, but careless tinting, bleaching, or permanent waving can result in broken and unsightly hair.

Hair coloring and permanent waving have become acceptable practices. In fact, psychiatrists and skin specialists agree that such cosmetic aids can do a great deal of good psychologically, since an individual's appearance has much to do with his mental health.

In spite of this approval, one significant fact should be noted: many people with dull, lifeless, and/or unmanageable hair (which may be thinning or graying) resort to coloring and permanent waving in an effort to make their hair more attractive; not only are their efforts usually in vain, but also such cosmetic practices may further enfeeble "sick hair."

While hair coloring and permanent waving are useful beauty aids, they do have their limitations. The answer to healthy hair is not found in a beauty shop.

Conclusion

Brushing, massaging, and shampooing are measures that every person can and should take because they help keep the hair and scalp clean and well groomed. In addition, they also aid in providing a healthy environment for normal hair growth. Each of these personal services should be performed regularly, preferably according to a fixed schedule, since human beings are creatures of habit. In themselves, however, they are not effective in checking baldness, grayness, dandruff, or abnormal oiliness. These are problems having deeper roots.

CHAPTER 3

Facts About Hair Products

In attempting to maintain or recapture youthful-looking hair, many of us reach out eagerly for anything that promises help. Knowing little about our hair and scalp, however, we are easy prey for unscrupulous promoters. They know from long and profitable experience that people suffering from thinning or graying hair will try almost anything, at least once.

The current promoters of questionable hair products are quite unlike the crude medicine men of years ago who audaciously peddled ridiculous contrivances to the unsuspecting public. Today, large reputable business firms are in this field and are much more sophisticated in their selling approach. They rely on the subtle skills of the gray-flanneled pitchmen of Madison Avenue advertising agencies to create a demand for their products while cleverly circumventing the restraints of Federal and state authorities and the common sense of a better informed public.

Hair Products and the Federal Government

The Federal government has partially assumed the role of protecting the American consumer from unscrupulous businessmen by passing legislation to restrict gross malfeasance. Principal among such legislation is Section Five of the Federal Trade Commission Act, which in its original form (1914) forbade "unfair methods of competition" and was amended in 1937 to forbid "unfair or deceptive acts or practices in commerce." This has been interpreted by the courts to mean that misrepresentation, false advertising, misbranding, and the like are illegal if they deceive or are harmful to buyers. As a result, the word "cure" has disappeared from the glowing advertisements that describe hair products. A new strategy of deception, however, has replaced the old. Ads are worded more cleverly, hinting but not stating, fashioned subtly so that buyers read into it their own hopes.

Be skeptical of such expressions as "aids," "checks," "helps," "relieves," fights," and "tends to alleviate." Such words may be used in television commercials and other advertisements to create a false impression about a product. For example:

> (This product) has been conclusively proven to alleviate unsightly dandruff in 99 per cent of the cases tested.

The underlined words are emphasized, creating the impression that this product has startling effectiveness. If challenged by the Federal Trade Commission, however, the promoter would be quick to point out that "alleviate" does not mean "cure," that only "unsightly" dandruff is alleviated, and that "99 per cent" refers not to the general public but merely to a private sampling.

Tonics, Lotions, Shampoos, and Rinses

Since dandruff afflicts an estimated 70 million Americans, it has received a large share of attention by hair-products promoters. By advertising extensively on radio and television, and in other media, they have succeeded in making dandruff as socially repugnant as body odor. The success of their campaign has set cash registers ringing cheerfully from Bangor to Palm Springs.

An imposing array of dandruff "cures" are promoted in the form of shampoos, rinses, lotions, and tonics.

(Actually, the term "hair tonic" is to be abandoned under the new law as meaningless and inaccurate.) Some of these products merely create the illusion of curing dandruff by unnaturally loosening deeper layers of cells; as soon as one stops using the preparation, the dandruff reappears. Other products do little more than wet down the dandruff flakes and prevent them from being shed so readily. In addition, it should be noted that ingredients in some of these preparations can irritate the scalp or have a drying effect that in the end intensifies the loss of skin cells.

In spite of their varying claims, it is an incontestable fact that hair shampoos, rinses, lotions, or tonics with or without antiseptics, vitamins, hormones, lanolin, or sulfa drugs are no more successful against baldness than they are against dandruff.

A well-known dermatologist was called forward in a Cleveland courtroom to give expert opinion. Asked whether or not there was any product that would stop excessive hair loss, the doctor smiled. If there were a successful remedy, he would have used it long ago, he said, adding that he had tried a multitude of products with results that were obvious. Everyone in the courtroom laughed, for the doctor was completely bald.

Outright Frauds

Some companies even go so far as to use false advertising deliberately, because they know that the Federal Trade Commission is hampered by too much work, too few investigators, and long legal delays. This allows some opportunists to push through a crash program, make a "killing," and back down when the Commission challenges them. It is an old saying that "a lie travels halfway around the world while the truth is still getting its pants on."

One such company announced that a germ called *Pityrosporum ovale* was the real cause of dandruff and rushed a new product onto the market that would rid the scalp of this germ. It sold briskly while the company stalled off the aroused Federal Trade Commission. After several months, however, the FTC forced the company to stop this line of advertising. Even so, the product had established a nation-wide reputation by this time, and the action by the FTC probably went unnoticed by the great majority of Americans. The company, meanwhile, rewrote its advertisements to imply a cure for dandruff without actually claiming one. And, although it complied with the FTC ruling, the company nevertheless remained in business, selling the same product to the unsuspecting average American.

Another swindle got off to a flying start some years ago when a company proclaimed that it had discovered a so-called antigray vitamin of calcium pantothenate and para-amino-benzoic acid which could restore hair to its original color. Not only was this miracle promised, but users of the new product were also told that they could expect to look and feel years younger. The company made a fortune before the Food and Drug Administration could definitely prove the whole thing a hoax.

Conclusion

In spite of all that has been written in this chapter, not all hair products on the market are useless. The important thing to determine is which products are worthwhile.

The answer to this question is not so complicated as one might think, as long as the buyer is not looking for miracles. For example, the main purpose of hair dressings is to aid in grooming; the product that best fulfills the individual need in this area is the one to buy. Other "built-in" attractions, such as dandruff or baldness deterrents, should be ignored. These are merely gimmicks dreamed up by advertising agencies attempting to stimulate sales.

The Federal Trade Commission should not be expected to stop deceptive advertising completely, even if their budget were greatly increased. False and misleading advertising will continue to exist in the hair-products field until the public learns the true nature of common hair and scalp problems.

CHAPTER 4

Hair and Scalp Clinics

In some respects, the most fraudulent activity involved with treatment of the hair and scalp concerns the hair and scalp clinics who advertise that they can stop baldness and dandruff and grow more virile hair. Several of these are now international in scope, having large offices in the major cities of the United States, Canada, and Europe. In addition, there are literally hundreds of small, independent clinics in large and medium-size cities throughout the country. Unwilling to leave any pocketbook unturned, some clinics send traveling "experts" into towns too small to support a full-scale operation.

As with the peddlers of useless hair products, the advertisements of these clinics are masterpieces of implication. Without directly stating it, they claim that their "exclusive" treatment can prevent, postpone, or correct baldness.

Most of these clinics support their claims by "evidence" of startling cures, using the familiar before-and-after pictures and testimonials. These deserve special explanation. First of all, the people pictured are real, and almost always they have experienced a regrowth of hair. A closer examination of their case histories, however, would bring out some interesting facts. Invariably these people are not victims of the type of baldness (common baldness) which accounts for the great majority of cases, but have *temporarily* lost their hair (baldness in patches or postinfectious baldness) as a result of severe shock, a high-fever illness, or some other acute disturbance. At some time during their period of misfortune, they attended a clinic for treatments. Subsequently the hair reappeared. The misguided victims, grateful for deliverance, are only too happy to praise the clinic's "cure" and permit their names and pictures to be used as "proof" to attract others. What they failed to realize is that in such cases it is unnecessary to resort to scalp treatments because regrowth of hair usually takes place naturally.

The Clinic "Treatment"

A visitor to a typical hair and scalp clinic finds the offices impressive. The staff generally consists of a manager who refers to himself as a "trichologist," an attractive receptionist, and several former hairdressers who administer the treatments. Everyone is usually dressed in a white uniform and, along with the antiseptic smell of a hospital in the air, a convincing medical atmosphere is created.

Interestingly, some of the clinics employ the services of a medical doctor. This became almost a necessity after one clinic was convicted of practicing medicine without a license. The added expense of employing a doctor has been put to good advantage by these clinics, however, because it has enabled them to advertise that their treatments are medically supervised and approved. The competence and the motives of such doctors are certainly questionable, but such a practice is not technically illegal.

On his first visit the "patient" is usually taken into a private inner office. Here the "trichologist" records the general information about the patient and the nature of his problem. During this ritual, time is provided for the patient to be impressed by a wallful of colorful charts and before-and-after pictures, together with a prominently displayed "certificate" of qualification.

It seems that these certificates must be issued by the company using them, since neither the American Medical Association nor any other qualified authority recognizes any lay specialist known as a "trichologist." The truth is that, as far as can be determined, he has no license or formal training in a qualified school of any kind. Anyone can call himself a "trichologist." The main individual requirements seem to be a full head of hair, a good sales personality, and a strong desire to make easy money. As for legal requirements, the only thing usually necessary to operate a hair and scalp clinic is to employ licensed hairdressers to administer the treatments. The "trichologist" hides behind the hairdressers' licenses; without them he would be little more than the arrogant medicine man who roamed the countryside during the horse-and-buggy era.

Once the paper work of the first visit is completed, the patron's scalp is examined under a lighted magnification lens, while the "trichologist" carefully parts the hair with different colored swabs. Then he glibly describes the "patient's hair problem," using a chart on the wall which shows an enlarged cross section of the scalp. If asked any questions by the patient, he has an impressive pseudomedical reply. And almost without exception he is sure to find the problem a serious or potentially serious one. Just as the patient is beginning to lose hope, though, the "trichologist" assures him that the clinic can solve his problem if treatment is begun at once.

Almost all hair and scalp clinics claim that it is their policy to refuse hopeless cases. This is a commendable gesture. By their standards, however, it seems that only a headless person would be labeled a hopeless case.

By far the most appealing item in the sales pitch of some clinics is the "written guarantee." It usually states that if, at the end of five treatments, the client is not satisfied with his progress, the money will be paid back in full. How could anyone resist giving this a try? Actually, the "trichologist" knows from experience that he can persuade almost all of the patients to continue their treatments beyond the expiration of the guarantee simply by assuring the client that progress is taking place beneath the surface of the scalp.

During the sales pitch the patient may be given a choice between clinic treatments and home treatments. The emphasis is put on the clinic treatments as being more effective. Naturally, they are more expensive. The average cost of a 40-clinic-treatment plan is about $200, with two or three treatments per week recommended. A home-treatment kit usually sells for about half as much for the same number of treatments. Regardless of the plan selected, the patient finds that an additional $25 or so will be required for a hair brush and special shampoos, solvents, and hair dressings (which must be repurchased from the clinic again and again, as they are used). In addition, some clinics sell "medicine" to be taken internally which is supposed to help make the external treatments more effective.

Of the many clinics, each claims that its particular approach is the answer. One stresses the use of antiseptics "to combat the germs and waste products." Another stresses stimulation "to rejuvenate cellular growth," while another claims that "nerves" are the villain and stresses soothing vibration apparatus.

The treatments are usually given in small, semipartitioned booths. So-called "secret formulas" of ointments, lotions, and sometimes shampoos are employed, along with some sort of massaging or plucking technique. Ultraviolet lamps, mechanical vibrators, high-frequency machines, heat lamps, suction cups, and other contrivances are used. Whatever the particulars, the complete ritual impresses most people, and hope replaces common sense.

Conclusion

It is difficult for most people to understand why such deceitful activities as these hair and scalp clinics are allowed to exist in this country. The Constitution, however, guarantees the right of free enterprise, and the clinics take advantage of this freedom. They infest our cities and get rich on money taken from men and women who are genuinely concerned about their hair and scalp. It is only natural for sufferers to turn to these quacks who set themselves up as authorities and imply the ability to effect cures.

While free enterprise should not be interfered with directly, there are other ways in which these charlatans can be suppressed. One way would be to make hairdressers' licenses unavailable to the promoters of these clinics, for without them they cannot legally operate in most states. This can be done through the hairdressers' and cosmetologists' associations, which can bring pressure to bear in the right places in order to restrain or prevent licensed hairdressers from working for these clinics. All the sincere members of these organizations should certainly lend their support, since this activity of a few of their cohorts is a discredit to their profession. Another way of eliminating this quackery is to replace ignorance with knowledge.

If all of the disappointed patrons of these clinics were willing to tell others of their experience, these clinics would not flourish. Being human, though, they are ashamed to admit that they have been "taken," and choose to suffer in silence. And there are probably some people who never even realize that they have been fooled.

Nevertheless, even if all the deceived victims were willing to pass the word around, this would not be enough. Sufferers will continue to seek relief from these quacks until a qualified authority substitutes in their place the proper approach to hair and scalp problems along with an effective explanation. The medical profession should be this authority. The next chapter shows why it has failed the general public in replacing fallacies with truths.

CHAPTER 5

Medical Doctors and Hair and Scalp Problems

As previous chapters have indicated, countless numbers of people resort to useless products, worthless scalp treatments, and other nostrums in efforts to combat hair and scalp problems. The prevalence of this quackery, along with widespread confusion and superstition, tends to confirm the fact that the medical profession has not asserted itself successfully in this field.

What is the position of the medical profession in regard to the more common hair and scalp problems? And why has it failed the general public in replacing fallacies with truths? To answer these questions is the primary purpose of this chapter.

Where the Position Is Clear

Dermatologists, who are physicians specializing in diseases of the skin and its appendages, can successfully treat most hair and scalp diseases. A list of these would include ringworm, favus, wens, baldness in patches, postinfectious baldness, and others. With diseases such as these, the issue is clear. Diagnosis and prognosis are usually plain and effective treatments available. Unfortunately, the hair and scalp problems that afflict the great majority of people fall not within this category but into one where the position of the medical profession is not so clear.

Where the Position Is Clouded

In contrast to the disorders just mentioned, the position of the medical profession with regard to common baldness, common grayness, and dandruff is clouded. Up to this time the medical profession has been unable to get across to the general public effective explanations of when these conditions are symptoms and when they are cosmetic problems — or, in other words, when something can be done about these problems and when not.

In the average case of thinning or graying hair, dermatologists propose no cure or treatment and urge the victim to accept the situation with as good grace as possible. In the average case of dandruff, dermatologists again propose no cure although they may prescribe medication to help *control* it. About the possible cause or causes of these conditions, they lapse into incoherent generalities.

All in all, statements made by medical doctors concerning common baldness, common grayness, and dandruff have filled the air with words which have produced more uncertainty than direction. The result: a gap has been created between the public and the medical profession concerning hair problems. Unfortunately, this needless gap has been filled by charlatans and useless products.

Conclusion

Those concerned want to know why they are losing their hair, why it is turning gray, why they have dandruff, or why they have oily, dry, lifeless, or unmanageable hair. And more important, they want to know the best method of combatting these problems. Until these questions are answered adequately, confusion and anxiety will prevail and superstition and quackery will flourish.

PART II

*Understand Hair and Scalp Problems;
Recognize Your Own Type*

CHAPTER 6

How Hair and Scalp Problems May Be Classified

Most books and articles on the subject present a bewildering variety of hair and scalp problems, and, unless the reader is familiar with the subject matter, it is almost impossible to untangle the ambiguities.

In an effort to avoid such confusion, this book divides hair and scalp problems into three categories: (1) treatable, (2) nontreatable, and (3) questionable.

In this chapter these categories are defined. In the chapters that immediately follow, the various types of baldness, grayness, and other common hair and scalp problems are described and placed in one of these categories.

Nontreatable Conditions

Nontreatable hair and scalp conditions are those which are so closely related to the physical makeup of a person that they can scarcely be considered disorders even though they may be unpleasant. Heredity is almost always the most significant factor. Examples in this category are kinky hair, congenital baldness, and congenital grayness. Abnormalities such as these are as characteristic of the person afflicted as is the color of his eyes. Unfortunately, there is no treatment which can permanently change any of these conditions.

Treatable Disorders

This category includes those disorders which can be effectively treated by a physician. It can be subdivided

Classification of Hair and Scalp Problems

Classification		Problem
Nontreatable Conditions		Congenital grayness (7) Congenital baldness (8) Common scurf (9) Common oiliness (10) Kinkiness (12)
Treatable	Scalp Diseases	True seborrhea (10) Ringworm (11) Favus (11) Dermatitis venenata (11) Traction baldness (8)
	Symptomatic Disorders	Accidental grayness (7) Postinfectious baldness (8) Baldness in patches (8) Dandruff* (9) Abnormal oiliness (10)
Questionable Problems		Common grayness* (7) Common baldness* (8)

* indicates problems about which this volume is mainly concerned.

(#) indicates the chapter in which the problem is described.

into (a) scalp diseases and (b) symptomatic disorders.

The first of these subdivisions includes such diseases as ringworm, favus, and true seborrhea. These local scalp conditions can be readily diagnosed and remedies prescribed. With proper medical supervision they can be cured.

Treatable symptomatic disorders include accidental grayness, postinfectious baldness, baldness in patches, and dandruff. Disorders such as these are symptoms primarily of a disease or some body imbalance. Diagnosis can be made by a physician and treatment prescribed, and normal hair growth, hair color, or scalp condition may be re-established.

Questionable Problems

Because in some cases they are treatable and in other cases they are nontreatable, common baldness and common grayness are separately classified as questionable problems. The determination of when they are treatable must be resolved on an individual basis. Fully explaining this point is perhaps the most important purpose of this book.

CHAPTER 7

Grayness

It has been estimated that 55 million people in this country have gray hair, and with the average life span continually increasing, this number seems destined to grow also. Although graying hair is probably not so disturbing a problem as baldness, there is evidence that many of those afflicted are genuinely concerned. According to one estimate, 60 per cent of the women with gray hair use an artificial hair coloring, and the number of men resorting to this device has been increasing rapidly.

Actors, actresses, and others employed in the entertainment and advertising professions are most concerned with this problem. They know that their careers often depend on their retaining a youthful appearance. On the other hand, there are some people in social and business life who actually prefer gray hair. They know that it usually lends distinction to their appearance and an aura of cogency. Often, in our paradoxical society, the young but gray-haired lawyer may carry more weight with the jury than his black-haired law-school roommate. Most people, however, would gladly trade their gray hair with anyone having naturally colored hair!

Strangely enough, true gray hair is relatively rare. What is frequently described as a head of gray hair turns out on closer examination to be a sprinkling of white hairs throughout more numerous dark brown or black hairs.

Gray hair is a condition known scientifically as *canities* (pronounced kah-NISH-eez). The three most common types are congenital grayness, accidental grayness, and common grayness.

Congenital Grayness

In the case of congenital grayness, the victim is born with white patches in his hair. The extreme form corresponds to complete albinism, in which there is a total lack of natural pigment in the hair or skin or both.

Fortunately, congenital grayness is a rare phenomenon. The cause has never been definitely determined, although heredity is usually considered to be the primary factor. Because the inherent defects are usually permanent, this condition is considered incurable.

Accidental Grayness

When graying follows severe physical or emotional shock, it is referred to as accidental grayness. It may occur in either sex, at any age, and develops over a relatively short period of time (as compared with common grayness). In some cases, this type of grayness may be only temporary, but generally it is permanent.

Included in this category are those legendary cases of individuals whose hair "turned white overnight." Marie Antoinette and Sir Thomas More are reported to have developed gray hair during the night before their execution. Lacking a scientific explanation for the sudden graying of hair, most authorities doubt the accuracy of such reports.

Common Grayness

By far the most common of the three major types of grayness is common grayness. This type of graying usually develops slowly but inexorably. As a rule, it begins at the temples and gradually sweeps backward across the top of the head. In other cases it develops evenly throughout the scalp until the hair is predominantly silvery gray or white. There are also instances in which the graying process develops unevenly, often leaving only the back part of the scalp its normal color.

Chronologically, common grayness is often first noticed in the early thirties, although in many instances it occurs earlier in life. More often it does not begin until the fourth decade, and it may be late in life before it develops fully.

An understanding of the nature of common grayness has eluded man ever since the dawn of civilization. While innumerable theories have been advanced, we are still faced with widespread confusion.

Actually, the world of science has, in recent years, determined the true nature of common grayness. To date, however, no attempt has been made to present to the public an explanation of these findings in their proper perspective.

It is now known that the development of common grayness is the result of certain aging changes that take place in the scalp tissue. These degenerative changes, which occur with advancing age, gradually diminish the activity of the cells responsible for the production of pigment.

In order to understand the true nature of common grayness, therefore, it is necessary to realize that it is directly related to aging. In this respect it occurs in the same manner as does wrinkling of the skin, redistribution of body weight, bent posture, and the failing of eyesight or hearing. All are caused by degeneration of tissue that occurs with advancing age, and can be regarded as "external characteristics of aging." It is the manner in which we grow old. Thus, the older we get, the grayer we can expect to become, until at some ripe old age all of our hair may be white. Nothing can cure common grayness, just as nothing can cure wrinkling or prevent us from growing old.

The explanation of the nature of common grayness cannot stop here, however, because two important questions remain unanswered: (1) why do some individuals develop common grayness at an earlier age than others? (2) why does the pattern of graying differ from person to person? The answers to these questions lead us to heredity: it is heredity that determines *when* the graying will develop, and the *pattern* in which it will manifest itself.

Unfortunately, nothing can be done to change the factor of heredity. It will be shown, however, that common grayness can unquestionably be checked, if it is developing prematurely.

Conclusion

The table on page 38 lists in their proper classification the three types of grayness presented in this chapter.

Congenital grayness is a nontreatable condition since it involves a permanent defect in the mechanisms that produce hair pigment.

Accidental grayness is a treatable symptomatic disorder because it is a symptom of a disease or some body disturbance. Once diagnosis has been made by a physician and treatment prescribed, normal hair color may return.

Common grayness is classified as questionable because in some cases it is treatable and in other cases it is nontreatable. The determining factor is whether or not it is developing prematurely.

Of the various types of grayness, this book is concerned mainly with common grayness. Part III will explain the role heredity plays and describe the actual aging changes that take place in the scalp as common grayness manifests itself. It will also be shown how this characteristic of aging can be checked if it is developing prematurely. In fact, in many cases, it may be possible to re-establish normal hair color and delay the onslaught of grayness for many years.

CHAPTER 8

Baldness

While the exact number of victims of baldness has never been determined in any generation, there is little doubt that baldness is prevalent today. Even the most casual observer is aware of this, particularly among adult males.

Baldness and its inevitable association with old age is by far the most distressing hair problem, especially in this country which is well known for its undue emphasis on youth.

Strictly speaking, only a completely hairless head should be called bald. For the purposes of this book, however, baldness will be referred to as any portion of a normally hairy scalp that suffers from hair loss.

Baldness is a condition known scientifically as *alopecia* (pronounced alo-PEESH-ya). What follows is a description of the five most common types: baldness from birth, postinfectious baldness, baldness in patches, traction baldness, and common baldness.

Congenital Baldness

Congenital baldness (baldness from birth) is a rare phenomenon. The victim may be born totally hairless or may be affected only on the scalp or on certain other body areas.

This type of baldness is often associated with faulty development of the skin, nails, and teeth. Although the cause has never been pinpointed, heredity is usually considered the primary factor.

Because the hair-growing mechanisms are in most cases either completely absent or permanently disabled, congenital baldness is considered incurable.

Postinfectious Baldness

Postinfectious baldness occurs when a loss of hair follows a siege of illness involving high fever. The high fever associated with such infectious diseases as influenza, pneumonia, and typhoid is known to be the cause of the resulting hair loss. The sustained fever produces toxins (poisons) which enter the blood stream and temporarily impair the functioning of the hair-growing mechanisms. Loss of hair may also occur after childbirth or a surgical operation and the impairing process may be similar.

Postinfectious baldness is usually characterized by diffuse hair fall over the entire scalp and generally occurs 60 to 90 days after the height of the fever or the birth of the child. Since the victim is already under the care of a physician in most cases, the reason for the hair loss can easily be determined. Once the general health of the body is or has been fully re-established, normal hair growth is nearly always experienced.

Syphilis is another common cause of postinfectious baldness. In its second stage, which occurs about six weeks to three months after infection, the hair begins to fall out rapidly. Total baldness is seldom the result; instead, the hair fall is scattered in intensity, leaving a moth-eaten appearance and a rash. After the disease is successfully treated, normal hair growth almost always resumes.

Baldness in Patches

In this condition the loss of hair may begin abruptly or gradually, leaving behind one or more small circular bald patches. As these patches become larger, they grow more oval, and the exposed skin becomes glossy and shiny. This condition is similar to ringworm of the scalp, except that there is a complete absence of hair stubs.

Baldness in patches follows no particular pattern. It may begin anywhere with a single patch and then be joined by other patches as the disease progresses. In its extreme form the entire scalp and body may be left without hair.

Rarely does the victim receive any warning of what is about to befall him. Some people recall having a severe headache. Then singly, or in large numbers, the patches appear.

Although much remains unknown about the fundamental cause of this disorder, certain types of severe

BALDNESS IN PATCHES

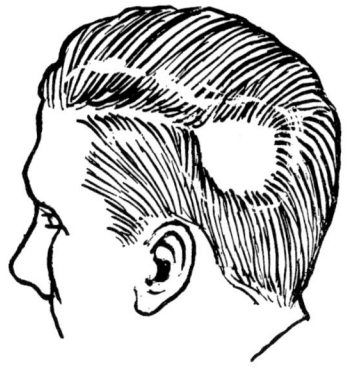

Typical early patch.

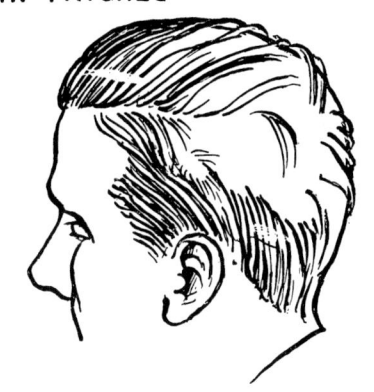

More extensive patching.

shock, fear, anxiety, or head injuries have been followed by this type of hair loss. People of all ages may become afflicted, male or female. Nervous individuals seem to be more susceptible to this disease than others.

Fortunately, regrowth of hair very often occurs. Regeneration is slow, however, and the first hairs are usually of the fine lanugo type. These may be permanent or subject to a second or third fall-out over the years before normal regrowth is established. When nonpermanent hair grows in, it reaches a length of about half an inch, then falls out. The hair that follows is thicker and longer and eventually returns to its normal color. Complete regrowth is more likely to happen in cases involving young people than with the middle-aged or the elderly.

Because baldness in patches could be a symptom of a serious body disorder, it is essential that a physician be consulted.

Traction Baldness

This type of baldness results from abusive pulling of the hair. It has been traced principally to the tightly drawn pony-tail hairdo, braids, and curling devices. The prolonged pulling caused by these practices is simply too much for some hair to endure. The scalp usually reacts to this punishment by becoming inflamed, either on the surface, where it can be detected, or below the surface, where it may escape detection. The spotty or straggly type of baldness that may result is usually temporary, unless the injurious practice is continued.

A less common but far more drastic form of traction baldness is brought about by a psychoneurosis called trichotillomania. This is an impressive term meaning an abnormal desire to pull the hair. An irregular bald patch is usually the result. Trichotillomania is not a true

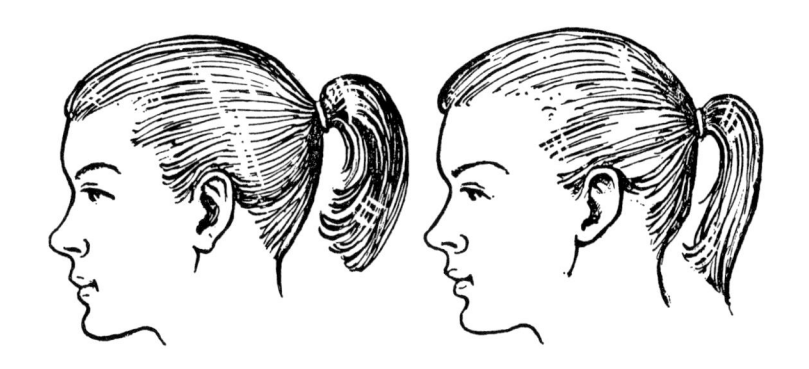

TRACTION (pony-tail) BALDNESS

form of insanity, but it is a common habit among the insane. In most cases the help of a psychiatrist is needed to stop it.

Baldness Due to Diseases of the Scalp

True seborrhea, ringworm, and favus are scalp diseases which usually result in loss of hair. In the interest of clarity they are discussed separately in Chapters 10 and 11.

Common Baldness

Common baldness accounts for over 90 per cent of all cases of baldness. There are two kinds: common unpatterned baldness and common male-pattern baldness.

Common unpatterned baldness is characterized by a diffused thinning that does not follow a recognizable pattern. It almost always occurs in women. At first the bald areas may hardly be noticeable, because the thinning is general and usually develops slowly. Excessive fall of hair may begin early in life, but usually the hair loss is not permanent until the fourth, fifth, or sixth decades. Hardly ever do women develop this diffused type of baldness to the extent that men develop their characteristic fashion of becoming bald.

Common male-pattern baldness, being much more prevalent, is already known to most people. As a rule, the loss of hair begins at the temples and, as the hairline gradually recedes, it forms the letter M. Simultaneously, a bald spot usually develops on the vertex of the scalp, and, as the hair loss continues, this bald spot expands and eventually meets the receding front hairline. The development of this pattern may vary slightly from person to person, but is nevertheless quite distinctive. In extreme cases only a fringe of hair around the base of the scalp survives. This type of baldness generally manifests itself earlier in life than the unpatterned type. It may begin in the early twenties, but generally does not develop fully until the third, fourth, or fifth decades.

Male-pattern baldness almost always occurs in men because a predominance of male sex hormones must be present before it will develop. In order to enable you to fully understand this point, a brief explanation of the relationship between hormones and hair follows.

Among the different systems of the human body (circulatory, digestive, respiratory, etc.), probably the one that the world of science knows least about is the endocrine system. This system is made up of several different glands, distributed throughout the body. These glands produce substances called hormones or "chemical messengers" which are secreted directly or indirectly into the blood stream. For this reason they are known as glands of internal secretion. Their chief work is maintaining the balance of the activities of the other systems of the body by increasing or decreasing their functioning.

The chief endocrine glands are the pituitary, thyroid, parathyroid, adrenals, and the sex glands (testes in the male, ovaries in the female). Each produces distinctively different hormones.

Because of their profound influence on the retention, distribution, growth, and regrowth of hair, only the sex hormones will be discussed in detail.

Although it is commonly assumed that men are better hair-growers, the male and the female have the same potential to produce hair on any part of the body where hair is normally found. Accordingly, there is not a single area which is hairy in men that may not become hairy in women under abnormal conditions.

Both male and female sex hormones are produced in each man and woman, and it is the relative quantity of each of these hormones that determines the distribution of hair on certain areas of the bodies of both sexes. These areas include the face, chest, shoulders, abdomen and back. Hairiness on these areas is a secondary male sex characteristic brought about by the predominance of male sex hormones. Since women ordinarily produce a minimal amount of male sex hormones, it is a secondary female sex characteristic to have an *absence* of hair on these same areas.

There are some common areas of hairiness in both men and women which are not under the control of the sex hormones. These areas include the fine, short, lanugo hair all over the body, the eyebrows and the eyelashes.

In the case of scalp hair, we are faced with something of a paradox. Whereas most of the body's hair growth is stimulated by male sex hormones, on the scalp the effect may be the reverse. In fact, a predominance of male sex hormones must be present before common male-pattern baldness can take place. This explains why women do not ordinarily develop patterned baldness. It seems that female sex hormones tend to encourage the growth of scalp hair and discourage the growth of body hair.

These facts are brought out vividly in the cases of men who were castrated before puberty or who never matured sexually. It was found that they developed very little body hair, and that which did grow was of the female type. In addition, there was little hairiness on their faces, but they often possessed heads of thick, healthy hair. Furthermore, such persons retained the straight hairline of a child and did not develop common male-pattern baldness, because the important male hormone-producing glands were either removed or remained infantile.

On the other hand, when such persons were given injections of male sex hormones, they developed early male-pattern baldness whenever this inherited characteristic was present.

The logical conclusion of these observations was the idea that male baldness could be cured by injections of female sex hormones. This has been tried, but with mixed results. The administering of female sex hormones to men invites changes in the body of a feminizing nature, as well as sterility, impotency, and other undesirable side effects. In an effort to minimize these side effects, researchers are presently experimenting with injections of various hormonal products directly into the scalp. To date, this approach has been proved practical only in efforts to grow eyebrows and hair lost in patchy baldness.

In rare cases a woman will develop the pattern of male baldness. This may indicate the presence of too many male hormones. In all such cases the individual should consult a medical doctor, since this may signify a serious bodily derangement.

In summary it must be noted that, while a predominance of male sex hormones must be present before male-pattern baldness will develop, these hormones do not represent the fundamental cause of the hair loss. If this were the case, all men of all racial strains would be bald. A predominance of male sex hormones merely determines that common baldness will manifest itself in the characteristic male fashion.

As with common grayness, the problem of common baldness of both types has baffled man through the ages. Literally hundreds of theories have been advanced, but these have been either invalid or incomplete. Only the wake of confusion remains.

Actually, the world of science has, in recent years, determined the true nature of common baldness. But heretofore no attempt has been made to present to the public an explanation of these findings in their proper perspective.

It is now known that the development of common baldness is the result of certain aging changes that take place in the scalp tissue. These degenerative changes which occur with advancing age gradually diminish the capacity of scalp tissue to produce long, soft hair.

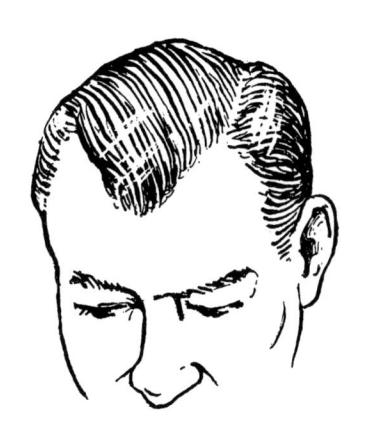

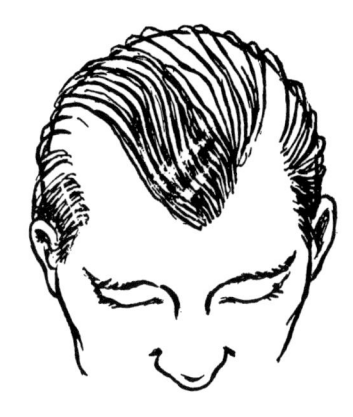

STAGES OF COMMON MALE PATTERN BALDNESS

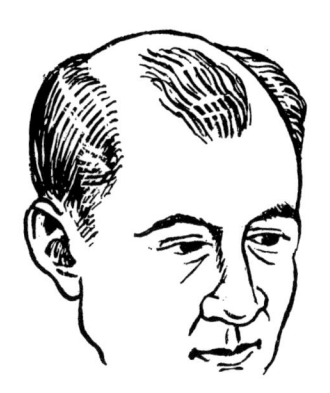

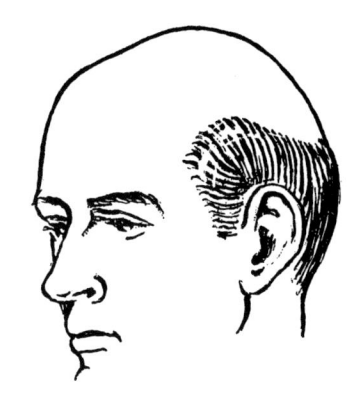

The primary fact we must realize, therefore, if we wish to understand the true nature of common baldness, is that, like common grayness, it is directly related to aging. It is an aging problem just as wrinkling of the skin, redistribution of body weight, bent posture, and failing eyesight and failing hearing are aging problems. All are caused by the degeneration of tissue that occurs with advancing age, and can be thought of as "external characteristics of aging." It is the manner in which we grow old. The older we become, therefore, the more hair we are likely to lose, until in old age—if we live that long — many of us will have little or no hair. Because this is a fact of life itself, nothing can cure common baldness, just as nothing can cure wrinkling or prevent us from growing old.

The explanation of the nature of common baldness does not stop here, however, because two important questions remain unanswered: (1) Why do some individuals develop common baldness at an earlier age than others? (2) Why does the pattern of hair loss differ from male to male, or female to female? (As already explained, it differs from male to female because of hormonal differences.) The answers to these questions again lead us to the subject of heredity. It is heredity that determines *when* the thinning will develop, and the *pattern* in which it will manifest itself.

Unfortunately, nothing can be done to change the factor of heredity. It will be shown, however, that common baldness can unquestionably be checked if it is developing prematurely.

Conclusion

The table on page 38 lists in their proper classification the five types of baldness described in this chapter.

Congenital baldness is nontreatable since it involves a permanent defect in the hair-growing mechanisms.

Both postinfectious baldness and baldness in patches are treatable symptomatic disorders, since either is a symptom that another disease or a body disturbance of some kind is or has been present. Once diagnosis has been made by a physician and treatment prescribed, total or partial hair growth may be re-established.

Traction baldness is considered a treatable scalp disease since it is a local condition which can be remedied.

Common baldness is classified as questionable because in some cases it is treatable and in other cases it is nontreatable. The determining factor is whether or not it is developing prematurely.

Of the various types of baldness, this book is concerned mainly with common baldness. Part III will explain the role heredity plays and describe the actual aging changes that take place in the scalp as common baldness manifests itself. It will also be shown how this characteristic of aging can be checked if it is developing prematurely. In fact, in many cases it may be possible to re-establish normal hair growth and delay the onslaught of baldness for many years.

(Much of the same phraseology was used to describe both common baldness and common grayness in order to emphasize that they are fundamentally the same type of problem.)

CHAPTER 9

Scaliness of the Scalp

Scaliness is the most common problem of the scalp. But, because it has never been explained to the public in its proper perspective, widespread confusion prevails.

Scaliness may present itself simply as a cosmetic problem (common scurf), or as an abnormal condition (dandruff).

Common Scurf

The top layer of the skin all over the body flakes off continually. These flakes are made up of dead cells, which were manufactured in a lower layer of the epidermis. This is a normal physiological process which enables us to renew our body covering. Most of this shedding goes on unnoticed because the minute particles are washed off or rubbed off by clothing or float away in the air.

The hair acts as a trap for these cells. Thus they are noticed on the scalp far more readily than anywhere else on the body. In some persons this shedding is normally more pronounced than in others, and they are described as having a tendency toward scaliness. It is normal for the predisposed individual and usually remains a personal characteristic throughout life. In any event, there is no reason for concern about this slight scaliness. It is only when an undue accumulation of this scurf occurs and is continually renewed despite ordinary brushing and shampooing that we have the abnormal condition commonly called dandruff.

Dandruff

Contrary to popular belief, dandruff is a disorder just as diarrhea is a disorder. It is an abnormal functioning of a basic physiological process. It may occur in either sex and appear, on and off, many times during a lifetime.

Three stages of dandruff can be distinguished. They are simple, compound, and eczematous:

1. Simple dandruff is characterized by an excessive and continual accumulation of small, loose, gray or white powdery scales. This flaking off of the upper layers of the epidermis is usually seen first in small, round patches. Part or all of the scalp may be affected. No inflammation or redness occurs, but itching is sometimes experienced. Usually the major distress is caused by the unsightly scales themselves when they become noticeable in the hair and on clothing. The question of when the scaliness is common scurf and when it is simple dandruff is best answered by the individual. What may be normal shedding to one person may be excessive shedding to another. The key indicator is the *change* in the degree of scaliness from one time to another.

2. Compound dandruff is a more serious stage. The scalp reacts to the excessive shedding by exuding a serum which grips the scales, making them adhere to the scalp in larger patches. The scales are not so easy to unseat as those in simple dandruff. They are waxy and yellow in appearance and later become almost crusted, although not greasy. Itchiness increases, and if some of the scaling is rubbed off, one notices a faint moisture and a slight pinkness of the underlying skin. This stage of dandruff may be mistaken for psoriasis, but the scales are thicker

and silvery in psoriasis and are usually not confined to the scalp area. If compound dandruff is neglected, it may sooner or later become eczematous. However, a more common sequel to compound dandruff is the supervention of true seborrhea (an infection of the sebaceous glands described in the next chapter).

3. Eczematous dandruff is basically compound dandruff which has become eczematous. The skin under the sticky, adherent scales becomes sensitized, and an eruption develops which looks red, moist, and raw. The affected scalp area may be small or fairly large, but its outer margin always seems to be irregularly circular. An inflamed rash may also appear on other parts of the body—for example, the ears, neck, brow, chest, or back. The itchiness is more severe than that experienced in the compound stage of dandruff; when the skin is scratched, the scales are loosened and bleeding or the oozing of serum may follow. This lays the scalp open to serious infection which further complicates the condition.

All three stages of dandruff are abnormal conditions and should be treated for what they are. Eczematous dandruff especially requires immediate medical attention in order to control the inflammation and guard against serious infection.

To date, however, the public has been led to believe that the basic problem of dandruff (the excessive shedding) is not an abnormal condition, that it is essentially a cosmetic problem like common scurf—merely a threat to poise and good grooming. As such, "remedies" have been concocted by cosmetic and pharmaceutical firms as well as medical doctors which merely control dandruff *symptomatically* without attempting to cure it properly—that is, *systemically*.

The fact is that dandruff is primarily a symptom of a body imbalance. Merely treating the symptom—the excessive scaliness — with special shampoos, ointments, and the like, will not remove the body imbalance which is causing it. The dandruff will persist, therefore, until the body imbalance has been counteracted.

Dandruff may be a symptom of one or more of a wide variety of body imbalances such as disorders in digestion and elimination, nervous system derangement, endocrine disturbance, and altered basal metabolism.

It is apparent, therefore, that the only effective way to cure dandruff is to determine the causative body imbalance in the particular case and to counteract it.

One school of thought had proposed the cause of dandruff to be a germ called *Pityrosporum ovale*. Although this micro-organism and others may be found on affected scalps and may be an aggravating factor, they do not represent the fundamental cause. Antiseptics, therefore, may kill any germs present, but they do not eliminate the cause of the excessive shedding.

In passing, it should be noted that, because dandruff is often accompanied by hair fall, it is apt to be considered the cause of baldness. This notion is entirely false.

Conclusion

The distinction was made between common scurf and dandruff, the former simply a cosmetic problem, and the latter an abnormal condition.

Common scurf is classified as a nontreatable condition because this slight scaliness represents normal shedding of the skin.

Dandruff, on the other hand, in any of its stages should be classified as a treatable symptomatic disorder since the excessive shedding is primarily a symptom of some body imbalance. Dandruff can be cured by detecting and effectively counteracting the causative body imbalance. Part III will show how more specifically.

CHAPTER 10

Oiliness of the Scalp

Oiliness is another common problem of the scalp. Here again, because this problem has not been explained to the public in its proper perspective, the issue is confused.

Oiliness may present itself simply as a cosmetic problem (common oiliness), as an abnormal condition (abnormal oiliness), or as a pathological condition (true seborrhea).

Common Oiliness

Within the skin all over the body are innumerable sebaceous glands. These tiny sacs secrete an oily substance called sebum, which helps keep the skin soft and supple and the hair lustrous. In some persons these glands are normally more active than in others, and as a result there is a tendency toward oiliness of the skin and hair. It is normal for the predisposed individual and usually remains a constant personal characteristic throughout life. While it may be an annoying cosmetic problem, there is no cause for concern. It is only when there is suddenly an abnormal amount of oiliness which continually renews itself despite ordinary washing that one has an actual disorder or disease.

Abnormal Oiliness

Abnormal oiliness, often referred to as seborrhea, is caused by an overstimulation of the sebaceous glands. It is characterized on the face by a shiny appearance and greasy feeling, and on the scalp it is readily detected by an unusual amount of oil on the hair. It is unlike common oiliness in that the individual afflicted may not have a normal tendency to oiliness, and the amount of oiliness varies, fluctuating from time to time between normalcy and profuseness. No inflammation or redness occurs, but itching is sometimes felt. Some hair fall may be experienced, but it is usually incidental. The major distress is caused by the greasy appearance and the difficulty in arranging the hair.

Like dandruff, abnormal oiliness is primarily a symptom of some body imbalance; it is not merely a cosmetic problem. Here again, in order to effect a cure, the condition must be approached systemically, by counteracting the causative body imbalance, rather than just symptomatically, as with special shampoos, ointments, and lotions.

True Seborrhea

True seborrhea is excessive oiliness accompanied by an infection of the sebaceous glands. It is much more serious than abnormal oiliness. Oiliness may be so pronounced that drops of oil form and have to be wiped off at frequent intervals. The scalp and other affected areas, which may include the face, especially around the nose and cheeks, the middle of the chest, and the spaces along the spine, flourish with micro-organisms. This pathological condition afflicts those almost always about or past the age of puberty. Men suffer more often than do women, although both sexes may have severe and lengthy attacks. This infection very often follows the compound stage of dandruff, giving its scales a greasier appearance.

The most serious consequence of true seborrhea is hair fall. Loss of hair usually begins over the crown and on the temples and is usually progressive if this condition goes unchecked; complete baldness results except for a fringe of hair around the base of the scalp.

True seborrhea requires immediate medical attention to combat the infection and check the loss of hair.

Conclusion

The distinction was made between common oiliness, abnormal oiliness, and true seborrhea. The first is simply a cosmetic problem and the latter two are abnormal conditions.

Common oiliness is classified as a nontreatable condition because a slight oiliness is the product of normally active sebaceous glands.

Abnormal oiliness, on the other hand, should be classified as a treatable symptomatic disorder since it is primarily a symptom of some body imbalance, as is dandruff. It can be cured by detecting and effectively counteracting the causative body disturbance. Part III shows how more specifically.

True seborrhea is classified as a treatable scalp disease since it is primarily a local infection of the scalp which can be successfully treated by a physician.

CHAPTER 11

Other Common Scalp Problems

Often an individual may have a nonspecific hair or scalp condition. There may be no sign of a scalp disease or graying; dandruff, abnormal oiliness, or excessive loss of hair may not be apparent.

The complaint may simply be that the hair is abnormally dry, dull, lifeless, or has a tendency to split.

These conditions are not discussed separately in this book, because they are basically the same type of problem as dandruff and often accompany it. When such conditions are not a result of inadequate care of the hair, they are symptoms of some sort of body imbalance. As with dandruff, once the causative body imbalance is effectively counteracted, the condition of the hair and scalp will almost certainly improve.

In this chapter three specific diseases will be discussed which are frequently encountered. The first two, ringworm and favus, generally result in loss of hair. The third, dermatitis venenata, is limited in its effects to varying degrees of inflammation.

Ringworm of the Scalp

Ringworm is a vicious disease brought about by a fungus (vegetable growth). It is highly contagious and may spread from animals to humans or from children to other children, depending on its type.

The human type is usually found in the scalp hairs of children who have not yet reached the age of puberty. This fungus is most commonly conveyed by the wearing of infected hats, caps, and clothing, and the use of towels and high-backed seats in theaters and conveyances. It begins as a small pink patch which becomes scaly as the disease progresses. One or more areas may be affected, and in extreme cases the entire scalp could be involved. The infected hairs become dry and brittle, lose their luster, and break easily on being pulled. The bald circular patches that usually result are covered with grayish scales, and around these patches can be observed stumps, redness, and dryness.

The animal variety, which is less common, is found in the scalp hairs of children, and in the nails, skin, and hairs of the bearded area of adults. Cats, dogs, and other domestic animals are usually the carrier of this fungus; transmission from one person to another is limited. It differs from the human type in that there is a certain amount of inflammation and pus formation present, and it heals much faster.

Early diagnosis and treatment by a competent physician is important to control the spread of the fungus. In most cases hair will grow again on the bald spots. If it is neglected, however, the hair follicles may be disabled, which results in permanent loss of hair.

Favus

Favus is another infectious fungus disease found primarily in the scalp. Unlike ringworm, this malady seldom strikes before puberty and is much less contagious. Either sex may contract it, but it is found most commonly in men.

Although one person may transmit the infection to another, animals are the principal carriers. Cattle, horses, dogs, cats, mice, fowl, and rabbits have all been known to spread the favus fungi. Fortunately, it is rarely encountered in epidemic form in the United States.

This fungus forms saucer-shaped, bright yellow crusts. It attacks the skin at the hair follicle, where it matures rapidly on the hair shaft and the skin. The odor of mice is characteristic when the yellow crusts are numerous. As the disease progresses, these crusts thicken, forming depressions in the scalp. The hair becomes dry and brittle and loses its luster. When the crusts have dropped off, the scalp is left hairless. Hair almost never grows again on the affected area. The aftermath of this disease results in favus scars, irregular glossy pink or white spots.

Early treatment by a physician is mandatory to prevent the spreading of the activity of the germ.

Dermatitis Venenata

This term covers all dermatoses that can be definitely traced to contact with drugs, or chemicals, or plant irritants. The skin of the scalp is often the site of the inflammation.

Dermatitis venenata is the correct technical term for so-called "hair dye poisoning" or "hair dye dermatitis," which occasionally follows the application of a certain type of hair coloring. Similarly, the various hair and scalp preparations, and any other substance which comes in contact with the surface of the scalp or other skin areas, may cause an inflammatory reaction.

Some of the drugs and chemicals which may be the villain are: bleaching powders; arsenic paints; caustic soda and potash; soaps and other detergents; insecticides, explosives, fertilizers, aniline and other coal-tar derivatives; salts of aluminum, copper, calcium, lead, and mercury; fur dyes (hair dyes); petroleum and its distillates (gasoline, kerosene, etc.); phenol, cresol, formaldehyde, resorcin and quinine (in scalp lotions); and pyrogallol.

Among the common plants which may cause dermatitis are: spruce, garlic, fennel, mustard, peppers, burdock, poison ivy, poison sumac, and ragweed.

The symptoms of dermatitis venenata vary greatly in different individuals, but to some degree redness, blisters, and itching are almost always present. Allergy (predisposition in the individual) is usually a prime factor. An idiosyncrasy may exist toward only one or toward several substances. Also, it may exist only at certain times, or when the system is otherwise upset from seemingly unrelated causes.

Victims of this condition may suffer from considerable fear and discomfort, but they can usually be assured of a complete cure. While the inflammation may require soothing medication, the important thing is to detect the offending substance and avoid it.

Conclusion

Ringworm, favus, and dermatitis venenata are classified as treatable scalp diseases since they are local conditions which can be successfully treated by a physician.

The scalp is subject to many other diseases, but these are beyond the scope of this book. In any event, a physician should be consulted for diagnosis and treatment.

PART III

Hair, Heredity, and Aging

CHAPTER 12

The Hair and Scalp and Aging

Sixteen of the more common hair and scalp problems have been described in the previous section. Hereafter, we are mainly concerned with only three of them: common baldness, common grayness, and dandruff.

The present chapter discusses briefly the nature of the hair and scalp. It explains how hair grows and gets its color, and how dandruff develops. And, perhaps more importantly, it describes the actual aging changes that take place in the scalp as common baldness and common grayness manifest themselves.

Of necessity, this chapter is more technical than the others in this book, but with the aid of the accompanying illustrations the average reader should have no difficulty in comprehending it.

The Skin (Scalp)

Hair, like nails, is composed of the same kind of cells of which the outer skin is comprised. In each case these cells cornify—that is, they change into dead, horny substance as they undergo a process known as keratinization. Thus we note the hardness of our nails, and under a microscope we find that horny, overlapping scales cover each hair. We see too that the outer skin of the body consists of innumerable flat scales which also overlap to form a tough, resistant, and practically waterproof covering for the entire body.

The outer layers of the skin are technically known as the epidermis. The epidermis consists of five stratified layers of cells. Each major layer of the epidermis differs from the others in the formation of its cells. The old cells of the top horny layer are shed or flake off continually as new cells created in the mucous or deepest layer of the epidermis are transformed into horny scales as they push toward the surface. By rubbing a portion of the body briskly, we can notice these tiny scales of dead cells. If, for some reason, this shedding becomes excessive on the scalp, we have the condition known as dandruff.

Just under the epidermis is the dermis, or true skin. It is composed mainly of a felted network of fibrous tissue and contains blood vessels, nerves, hair follicles, sweat glands, and sebaceous glands. The various tissue structures which the dermis comprises receive a continual supply of nourishment from the blood stream. Much of this vital nourishment is received in the papillae of the dermis—tiny nipple-like upward projections of the tissue just below the epidermis. These papillae exist in great numbers all over the body. Within the papillae are tiny blood vessels, called capillaries, which exude a serum. This serum seeps into tiny intercellular spaces of the epidermis and serves as its source of nourishment.

Below the dermis a third layer of tissue, referred to as the subdermis or subcutaneous layer, links the dermis with the tissue covering the muscles and bones. This layer contains many fat lobules and the main nerve trunks and blood vessels of the skin, as well as the larger sweat glands and the longer hair follicles.

The Hair and Allied Structures

Although hair is very much like the other appendages of the skin, its structure and growth are unique. There are three principal types of hair: (1) long, soft hair, such as that of the scalp, beard, pubes, and armpits; (2) stiff,

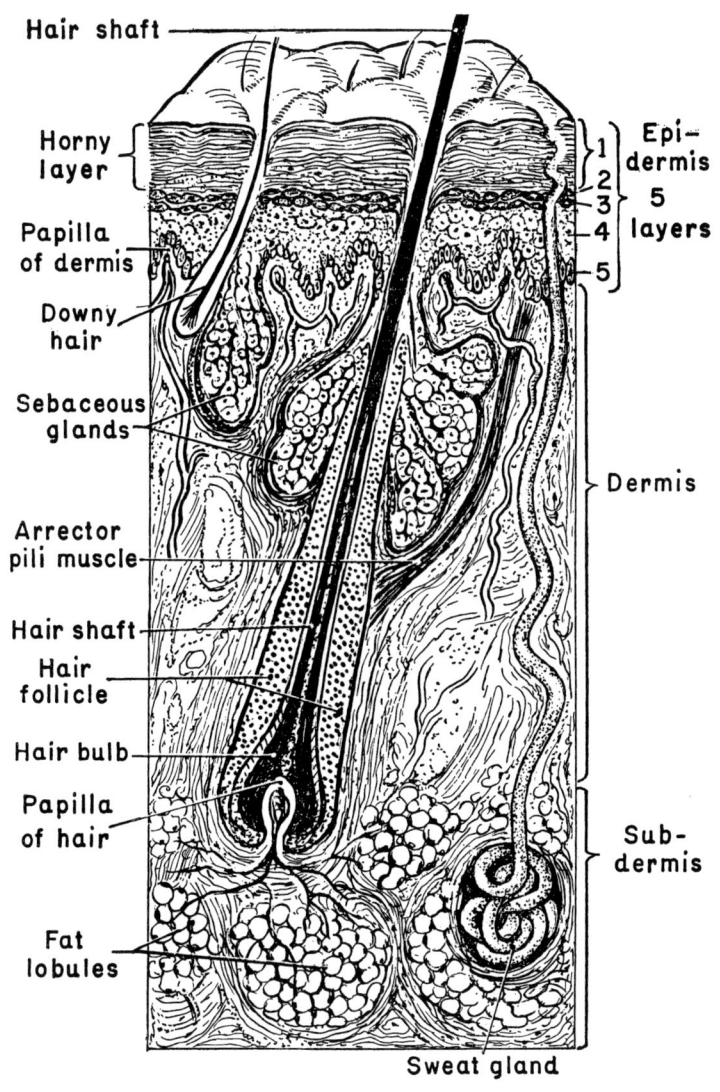

CROSS SECTION OF THE SCALP.

short hair, such as that of the eyelashes and eyebrows; and (3) fine, short lanugo hair, which is found over almost the entire body.

The average adult scalp holds 120,000 hairs. The finer the hairs, the more numerous they are. Blondes average about 140,000 hairs, brunettes about 100,000, and redheads about 90,000.

Each scalp hair emerges from a long narrow pocket in the skin called a follicle. At the bottom of the follicle is a nipple-like projection of tissue, the hair papilla. Like the papilla of the dermis, it contains capillary blood vessels. This is, however, a special type of papilla, because it is able to build hair.

The hair itself consists of thousands of the same kind of cells which make up the surface of the skin. But instead of forming into flat scales, these cells unite in the hair bulb (an inverted bowl-shaped growth of cells over the papillae) and are fused together into a long spine, as growth forces them upward through the narrow tube of the follicle.

Valuable allies of every growing hair are the sebaceous glands which are present in the skin all over the body except the palms of the hands and the soles of the feet. These small sac-shaped bodies enter the upper part of the follicle through a short duct. They secrete an oily substance called sebum which lends sheen and luster to the hair and helps keep the skin soft and supple. When the activity of these glands is hindered, the result is stiff, rough, and dry skin and hair. On the other hand, when the sacs are abnormally active, both skin and hair become excessively oily.

Directly below the sebaceous gland, a network of nerves surrounds the hair follicle. It is now believed that nerve endings also enter the hair papilla. The hair itself, however, contains no nerves, thereby explaining the reason why we feel no pain when our hair is cut.

To the side of each follicle of long, soft hair is attached a tiny involuntary muscle called the arrector pili, which contracts when we are frightened or chilled and causes the hair to "stand on end." These muscles are phylogenetic remnants and serve no purpose.

The hair length from the bulb to its tip, is called the hair shaft. It serves as adornment and protection and has elastic qualities which permit the hair to be stretched about one fourth its natural length. This prevents the hair from breaking easily when combed or brushed and makes possible the process of permanent waving.

There are three distinct forms of hair—straight, wavy, and kinky. Each is determined by the shape of the follicle from which it emerges. Straight hair grows from follicles

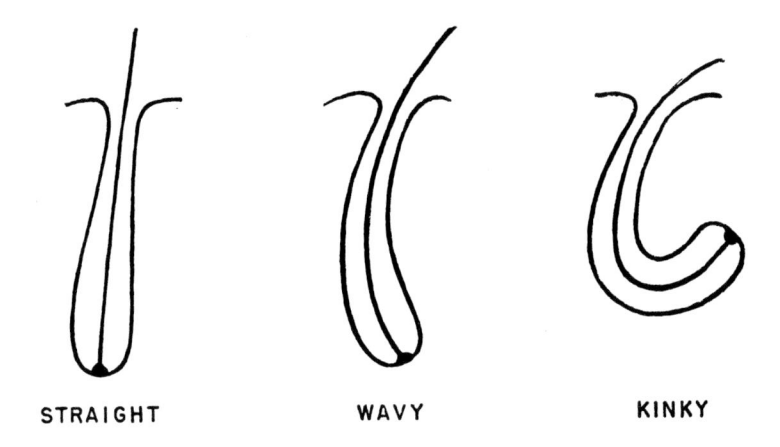

STRAIGHT   WAVY   KINKY

that are straight throughout their length, wavy hair from follicles that are slightly curved, and kinky hair from follicles that are sharply curved. In cross section straight hairs are round, wavy hairs are oval, and kinky hairs are

| STRAIGHT | WAVY | KINKY |

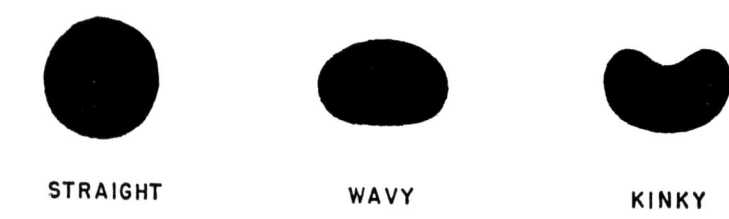

flat or kidney-shaped. Straight hair is most characteristic of the Mongolian and the American Indian, wavy hair of the Caucasian, and kinky hair of the Negro. (A multitude of products have been sold to straighten kinky hair, but the results are only temporary, since no treatment can change the shape of the hair follicles.)

When hair absorbs moisture from the atmosphere, it becomes longer and wider. As a result, naturally curly hair becomes more curly in damp weather, whereas straight hair, artificially curled, tends to straighten out again.

Although a full-grown hair looks relatively simple in appearance, it is actually composed of three distinct layers. The innermost or center layer, called the medulla, is made up of loose cells and some grains of pigment. This is surrounded by a thick cortex layer, which is made up of long, spindle-shaped cells that adhere to each other and give the hair its amazing elasticity and flexibility. This layer also contains the pigment which determines the hair color. The outside layer, known as the cuticle, protects the cortex. It is composed of flattened horny scales which overlap one another. These transparent scales grip the inside imbricated wall of the follicle securely and help prevent the hair from being pulled away from the papilla. Another purpose of the cuticle layer is to hold some of the sebum secreted by the sebaceous glands, thereby giving hair its luster and helping to pro-

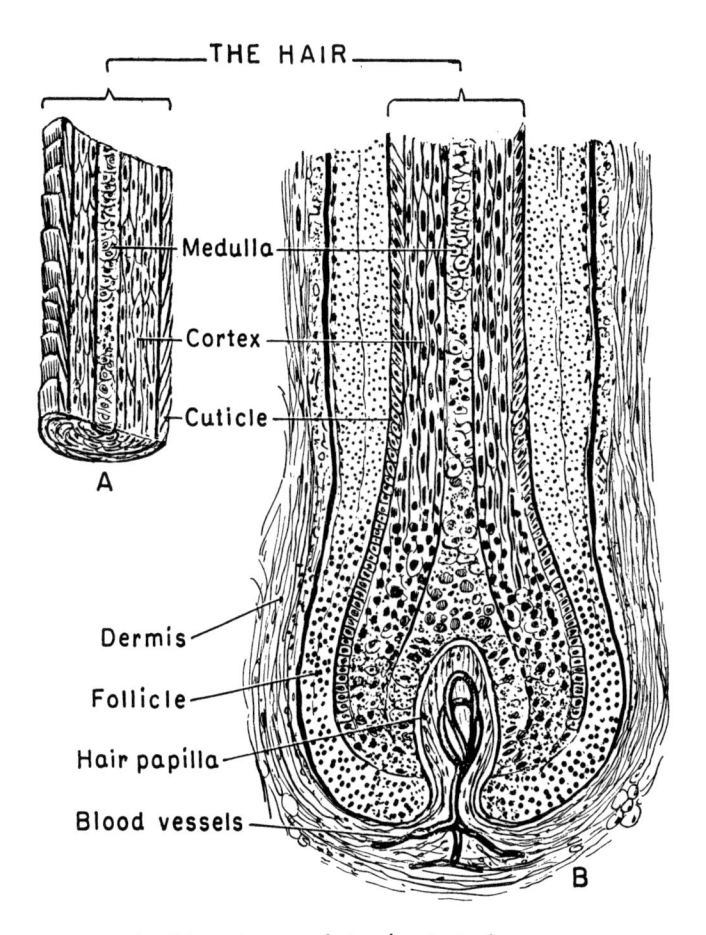

A. Structure of typical hair.
B. Hair in a follicle.

tect it from extreme weather conditions and harmful external agents.

Hair Color

Although superficial examination of hair would indicate a wide range of color hues, microscopical examination has revealed only three types of pigment: black, brown, and yellow. The final shade of the grown hair shaft is determined by the arrangement and varying proportions of the three. Color tones are also influenced by tiny air spaces present in and between the layers of the hair.

Pigment that colors hair is produced when the enzyme tyrosinase acts as a catalyst upon tyrosine, an amino acid. This activity occurs within the hair papilla and hair bulb as the hair grows.

When there is a deficiency of pigment in the hair shaft, it appears gray; when there is a complete absence of pigment, the hair shaft appears white.

Normally, the grayness of a hair starts at its bulb. Contrariwise, hairs may be found which are dark near the scalp and gray at the tips. Such an exception, however, is probably due to nothing more than the pigment-producing activity in the hair bulb becoming rejuvenated.

Growth and Loss of Hair

Scalp hair grows at a rate of about one-half inch per month. It grows faster in women than in men, faster during summer months than winter, and faster during daytime than at night. It is also interesting to note that the growth of scalp hair is generally fastest between 15 and 30 years of age and declines between 50 and 60 years.

In spite of the fact that a certain number of hairs are lost every day, the scalp tends to maintain a full crop of hair. This is because hair that has been shed is ordinarily replaced by new hair.

A scalp hair may "live" as long as seven years. During its life span, distinctive changes take place below the surface of the scalp in the shape of the follicle and the hair shaft. These changes occur in three distinct stages, commonly referred to as the "hair cycle."

This cycle starts with an active growing stage, which is followed by a transitional stage, characterized by a cessation of active growth, and ending with a resting stage. The cycle starts all over again, even before the old hair is shed, with the formation of a new hair from the same follicle. A detailed description of the exact changes that occur in the hair and scalp during the hair cycle is unnecessary for our purposes.

The length of the hair cycle, as well as the length of the stages within the cycle, varies in different follicles and in different areas of the body. Scalp hairs boast the longest cycle, 18 months to seven years, but have a very short resting stage. Hairs on other parts of the body have an average life cycle of only six months, but have a relatively long resting stage.

The scalp hairs in women have a longer life cycle than in men. This is one of the reasons why the hair of women grows to a greater length. It is also interesting to note that hair "born" during the summer has a greater life span and grows to a greater length than "winter hair."

Normally, as pointed out above, the hair cycle repeats itself, and so the rate of hair replacement tends to keep pace with the rate of hair loss. Obviously, hair loss is considered excessive only when the number of hairs shed is greater than the number of hairs replaced.

Excessive shedding or baldness occurs when the normal environment in which scalp hair grows is altered, or merely when the hair cycle of many follicles is adversely affected. A number of factors may be responsible, some of which have already been discussed. At the moment, however, we are concerned primarily with baldness brought about by changes in the scalp due to aging.

Aging of the Scalp

As we all know, none of us is immortal. With aging, the tissues of the body deteriorate, some more quickly and to a greater extent than others. Scalp tissue is not immune to this deterioration, and the result sooner or later is common baldness and common grayness.

Common grayness is the result of certain aging changes that take place in the cells of the hair papilla and hair bulb. These atrophic changes diminish the enzymatic activity responsible for the production of pigment. As a result, hair grows from the scalp deficient in pigment and appears gray. As the aging process continues, further degeneration may completely disrupt this pigment-producing activity, and the result is white hair. This regressive transformation may occur with or without loss of hair.

With reference to common baldness, the normal growth and regeneration cycle of scalp hair is inhibited by aging, and strikingly distinctive atrophic changes occur in the scalp tissue, causing baldness to some degree. A list of these degenerative changes follows:

1. The epidermis becomes thin.

2. The waviness of the junction between the epidermis and the dermis flattens.

3. The capillary blood vessels in the papillae of the dermis wither away.

4. The network of blood vessels and nerves of the dermis deteriorates.

5. Fatty tissues harden and shrink.

6. Scalp follicles producing long, soft hair undergo a regressive transformation into the lanugo type which are only capable of producing short, fine hair.

Individual hormonal differences (Chapter 8) and hereditary differences (Chapter 13) cause variation in these aging changes.

As we suffer hair loss and/or grayness due to aging, we can only imagine these dramatic degenerative changes occurring within the scalp. Much more apparent are the changes in the superficial appearance of the hair and scalp. Familiar to all of us is the fine, ghostly white hair of the aged, and the leathery, often shiny, appearance of the bald scalp.

When baldness or grayness occurs without this degeneration or some sort of permanent damage, as is usually the case in baldness in patches, postinfectious baldness, traction baldness, and probably in many cases of accidental grayness, hair growth and hair color may be reestablished, because the hair-growing and pigment-producing apparatus is potentially operative.

Conclusion

After all of these points have been made, it seems almost redundant at this point to add that hair is dead cellular matter. An end product of the body, it has no nerves, arteries, or muscles. It is one of the body's strangest and least understood phenomena. It appears to grow like a plant, and yet, when fully mature, it is discarded like waste matter. It reacts swiftly to emotions and the weather but can be cut to skin level without pain. Thoughtlessly, many of us spend more time trying to improve its appearance than we spend tending the health of the rest of the body.

The nature of hair may be more fully appreciated when it is considered as an integral part of the whole physical being; it is not an external, independent appendage of the body. Like the skin, hair may be considered a barometer of health in many individuals. When the body is in good health, the hair usually reflects this by being strong and lustrous. If the body's health is below par, the hair often responds by becoming dull, lifeless, and less elastic.

This chapter spotlighted a discussion of the actual aging changes that take place in the scalp as common baldness and common grayness manifest themselves. In order to learn when and why these two characteristics of aging are developing prematurely, the subject of heredity must be considered next.

CHAPTER 13

Heredity and Hair

Generally speaking, the formation of our makeup as human beings takes place between conception and maturity, and the degeneration of that makeup between maturity and death. During the formative phase of the life cycle, muscles, bones, nerves, and other tissues that make up the organs and systems of the body are developed. During the degenerative phase of the life cycle, our tissues deteriorate, causing the various characteristics of aging to manifest themselves, such as wrinkling of the skin, failing eyesight, failing hearing, as well as common baldness and common grayness.

While all of us grow up and grow old in a fashion which is similar, no two of us do either of these things in exactly the same manner. The basic cause of these individual differences is heredity.

This chapter deals mainly with the relationship of heredity to characteristics of aging, especially common baldness and common grayness. While these characteristics of aging result from degenerative changes that take place in scalp tissue, it will be shown that heredity plays a leading role because it answers why the pattern in which common baldness and common grayness manifest themselves differs from person to person and why some persons develop these characteristics of aging at an earlier age than others.

Individual Differences Due to Heredity

Scientists, as well as poets, have been amazed at the fact that no two people in the world—or, for that matter, in the entire history of mankind—are exactly alike. In spite of the fact that the birth experience is much the same everywhere, newborn infants begin to show signs of individuality almost immediately. Furthermore, the process continues without abatement throughout life.

The fundamental cause of this phenomenon is heredity.

Individual differences due to heredity are apparent in three general areas: physical characteristics, temperament, and intelligence. We observe that almost all of us have the accepted number of physical organs, but these differ in size, shape, color, and strength. We observe people to be big-boned, small-boned, tall, short, well proportioned, poorly proportioned, and we note the infinite gradations within these extremes.

In addition to these obvious physical differences, our temperament (why we think, feel, and act differently in a specific situation or in our social environment in general), and our intelligence (the kind of brain we are born with and the growth it experiences) are also inherited characteristics, for the most part.

These and a thousand other characteristics are packaged in tiny rod-like mechanisms called chromosomes. In conception 24 chromosomes from each parent are joined. Carried on these chromosomes are the genes which are the hereditary determiners. As cells divide to form muscle, bone, nerves, and other body tissues, the genes determine the particular characteristic of these tissues — for example, the particular color of eyes, the particular shape of the nose, the particular color and form of hair.

The genes function in pairs, one from each parent. Both are concerned with the same characteristic although the stronger one usually predominates in determining the particular formation of that characteristic.

Once our genetic makeup has been established, it cannot be changed. And, except in the case of identical twins (which begin life as one fertilized egg), no two persons can possibly inherit the same combination of genes. It is for this reason that each of us differs fundamentally from all other human beings. It also explains the similarities among members of the same family, since their genetic makeup is usually more similar than is that of unrelated individuals.

For the purpose of this book, we are primarily interested in genetic makeup with regard to the physical characteristics of aging.

Heredity and Characteristics of Aging

Most of us have probably never realized that the genes we inherit not only determine the pattern formation of our makeup but also determine the pattern of degeneration of that same makeup, resulting in a particular pattern of wrinkling of the skin, redistribution of body weight, bending over of posture, failing eyesight, and so on. This also holds true for our hair. Not only are the distribution, density, texture, and color of our hair determined by the genes we inherit, but also the eventual pattern of degeneration of scalp tissue resulting in (among other things) grayness and hair loss—common grayness and common baldness.

Thus the genes we inherit not only determine how we grow up but also how we grow old.

The fact that the manner in which we grow old is inherited is made unmistakably clear when we consider the comparison of identical twins. It is found that identical twins not only look alike in youth, when even parents have difficulty in telling them apart, but also look alike in old age. The pattern of wrinkling of the skin in various body areas remains the same, along with the manifestation of other characteristics of aging, including the pattern of graying and hair loss. Not only does the pattern remain the same, but also, the age at which the characteristic of aging develops tends to be duplicated. Since identical twins have exactly the same genetic makeup, the fact that the genes we inherit not only determine the pattern formation of our makeup but also the eventual pattern of degeneration becomes obvious.

If we wish to determine in ourselves the particular fashion in which the characteristics of aging will manifest themselves, we can get a reasonably good idea by observing older members of our family. Certain generalizations can be made regarding the physical characteristics of a particular family. We cannot, however, be certain of the exact fashion in which these characteristics will develop in ourselves, because there is only a similarity and not a duplication in the genetic makeup among members of one family. Only if it were possible to observe an identical twin of ourselves who had already grown old, could we conclude with any certainty how and when the characteristics of aging would manifest themselves in our own person.

Whatever pattern of aging we inherit we must accept. As pointed out earlier, our genetic makeup is irrevocably fixed at conception. Note, however, that an important factor in the development of our inherited characteristics is environmental exposure, which may modify them to some degree. Because environment is a variable and can be controlled by each of us to some extent, an important fact emerges. *Although we cannot change our individual aging characteristics, we can prevent them from developing prematurely, and this includes common baldness and common grayness.*

Environment Plays a Part

By environment is meant the aggregate of all the external conditions and influences affecting the life and development of an individual — for example, nutrition, climate, upbringing, education, and occupation.

Some individual characteristics, such as eye color, develop almost entirely uninfluenced by environment, and may therefore be referred to as characteristics which are hereditary. At the other extreme are those characteristics, such as the language we speak, which depend almost entirely on the environment in which the individual is reared, and may therefore be referred to as acquired. Most individual characteristics, however, result from a greater interplay between hereditary and environmental factors. A person's physique, for example, which is fundamentally an inherited characteristic, may be modified considerably by such environmental factors as diet and occupation. Similarly, intelligence may be modified by opportunities to observe and learn, while temperament may be modified through relationships with others.

Environmental exposure may also modify the development of aging characteristics. Various environmental factors, such as poor diet, emotional tension, and lack of rest and relaxation, may cause some people to grow old before their time. Whenever this happens, the characteristics of aging tend to manifest themselves sooner than need be. Thus, we have common baldness and common grayness, along with other characteristics of aging, manifesting themselves prematurely.

The fact that characteristics of aging can develop prematurely is made unmistakably clear when we again consider the comparison of identical twins. As stated earlier, identical twins look alike not only in youth but also in old age. Differences, however, do develop, some of which may be reflected in the signs of aging. While the general pattern of aging remains the same, it may appear obvious that one twin is developing the same characteristic of aging sooner than the other. Whatever differences do exist between identical twins must be attributed to environment since they have exactly the same genetic makeup.

You may, for example, be predisposed to begin developing common grayness at age 42. Common sense would dictate that this characteristic of aging in you would tend to manifest itself sooner if your physical resources were being constantly undermined by such environmental factors as poor diet, overwork, excessive smoking, and so on. While the body can function under all sorts of conditions, it will operate most efficiently under rather limited conditions.

Therefore, while heredity is the predominant factor in determining how we grow old, environment undeniably plays a part. Unfavorable environmental factors may cause the characteristics of aging to develop prematurely.

Premature Common Baldness and Premature Common Grayness

As previously mentioned, there are two types of common baldness: common male-pattern baldness and common unpatterned baldness. An important difference must be noted here.

As a rule, common male-pattern baldness develops at an earlier age than common unpatterned baldness or common grayness. It is not uncommon to observe men who have fully developed male-pattern baldness by age 30 or 35. In such cases we cannot necessarily conclude that these men have grown old before their time—that this particular characteristic of aging in them has developed prematurely. This may or may not be true, depending on their individual genetic makeup. The problem is to determine whether or not common baldness or common grayness is developing prematurely.

The terms "premature baldness" and "premature grayness" have in the past been used loosely. The result has been confusion and misunderstanding. The baldness in a 30-year-old person, for example, is referred to as "premature baldness" only because it has developed sooner than most people develop this condition. It may, however, be normal for some individuals to become bald by the time they are 30 years old. "Premature baldness" or "premature grayness," in the strict sense, occurs only when it has developed prematurely in a given individual.

Why common baldness and common grayness were not originally classified as either treatable or nontreatable can now be more readily understood. They are nontreatable *per se* because they are characteristics of aging which cannot be cured, just as growing old cannot be cured. There are, however, certain conditions, such as poor diet, emotional tension, and so forth, which can cause a body imbalance and result in the premature development of the aging characteristics. Since poor diet, emotional tension, and the like are environmental factors which can be corrected, *premature* common baldness and *premature* common grayness are treatable. More specifically, they should be classified as treatable symptomatic disorders, since their *premature* development is a symptom of some body disturbance which can be remedied.

But what about dandruff? Where does it fit into the picture? Dandruff is not a characteristic of aging like common baldness and common grayness. It is, however, exactly the same type of problem as *premature* common baldness and *premature* common grayness in that all are symptoms of some body imbalance.

Conclusion

All of us grow up and grow old. But because of hereditary differences, no two persons (except identical twins) grow up or grow old in exactly the same fashion.

Whatever pattern of aging we inherit must be accepted because our genetic makeup is fixed at conception. Certain conditions or environmental factors, however, can adversely affect our makeup and cause the characteristics of aging to develop prematurely.

If we wish to determine whether or not our own characteristics of aging are developing prematurely, we would only be speculating if we compared ourselves with other persons of the same age, because the genetic makeup differs in each of us. Even within our own families there may be a great range of differences. Only if we had an identical twin with whom we could compare ourselves would we be able to conclude with any degree of certainty whether or not we were aging prematurely. And even with this advantage, our conclusion could still be erroneous, since the twin might be growing old before his time.

How, then, can one determine if the characteristics of aging, and common baldness and common grayness in particular, are developing prematurely? This question will be answered in the next chapter, "Are You Growing Old Before Your Time?"

CHAPTER 14

Are You Growing Old Before Your Time?

We observed in the previous chapter that common baldness and common grayness are characteristic of aging, and that heredity determines for the most part when and how they will develop. It was also pointed out that we cannot prevent them from manifesting themselves, just as we cannot prevent ourselves from growing old. It has been stressed, however, that they can be checked if they are developing prematurely.

How, then, can one determine whether or not they are in fact developing prematurely?

Full Health and Disease

Of one thing we can be sure. Common baldness, common grayness, and other characteristics of aging will not develop prematurely if we are in full health.

If, on the other hand, a disease is present which is undermining the body's resources, it is reasonable to assume that the characteristics of aging are developing sooner than called for by the individual's makeup. In such cases premature common baldness and premature common grayness can be checked and possibly reversed if the disease is cured and full health restored.

Nevertheless, some persons develop common baldness and common grayness prematurely without the presence of a recognizable disease. In such cases a person can literally be growing old before his time without realizing it.

When an individual becomes gray or bald around age 40 or 50 without the presence of a recognizable disease, it is almost always considered an ordinary case of common baldness or common grayness. Rarely is it referred to as being premature, merely because there are so many people gray or bald at these ages. If no disease is present, a person who approaches a medical doctor might be told that heredity was the cause of his condition and that he should accept his fate with as good grace as possible. If the truth were known, however, we would no doubt be shocked by the number of cases of baldness and grayness that are blindly attributed to heredity but are actually premature developments of the aging process which could have been checked or reversed.

If we were to observe carefully the human beings with whom we come in daily contact, we would no doubt discover many excellent examples of common baldness and common grayness developing prematurely without the presence of a recognizable disease.

It is therefore apparent that, while being in a state of disease can cause common baldness, common grayness, and other characteristics of aging to develop prematurely, there is an area between full health and disease in which they may also be occurring prematurely.

The Twilight Zone of Health

While the body can function under a wide range of conditions, we are so constituted that it operates most efficiently under a rather rigid set of conditions. It is therefore possible to be free from disease and still not be in a state of full health.

Between the extremes of full health and disease we have what may be referred to as "the twilight zone of health." This is a state in which we cannot be considered healthy within our potential, nor can we be considered diseased by all practical standards.

We may be living in the twilight zone of health because of such causes as these:

A

Unbalanced diet	Excessive smoking
Vitamin deficiency	Excessive drinking
Mineral deficiency	
Overeating	Lack of rest and relaxation
Undernourishment	Lack of exercise
Food allergy	Overwork
	Excessive study
Anxiety	
Guilt	Miscellaneous allergies
Grief	
Dissatisfaction	

Any one of these may be the villain, but more often a combination of them causes the below-par state of health. Deficiencies, excessiveness, foolishness, and idiosyncrasies of this sort can cause such minor body imbalances as these:

B

High blood pressure	Altered metabolism
Low blood pressure	Nervous system derangement
Anemia	Blood sugar instability
Digestion disorder	Kidney disturbance
Elimination disorder	Acidosis
Endocrine disturbance	

These cannot be considered full-blown diseases, but they, too, undermine the body's resources just as surely.

For example, a perfectly healthy individual may become afflicted with anxiety (emotional tension), and develop a case of high blood pressure. Because a body imbalance is present, this person cannot be considered in full health. On the other hand, he cannot, in the strict sense, be considered in a state of disease, either. He finds himself in a state of health somewhere between the two. This is the twilight zone of health. The high blood pressure will persist (and possibly grow worse), and he will therefore remain in this gray zone until the underlying cause, the anxiety, is eliminated. While this high blood pressure condition may not affect him as acutely as a full-blown heart disease, it can just as surely undermine his body's resources.

Usually, when the general health of the body is affected, the hair and scalp are also affected. As indicated in a previous chapter, the hair and scalp of many individuals can be considered a barometer of health. Even slight body disturbances may be reflected by a change in the appearance of their hair and scalp.

Accordingly, the result of living in the twilight zone of health can cause common baldness and common grayness, as well as the other characteristics of aging, to develop prematurely just as disease can. This is especially true when minor body imbalances, such as those listed above, are allowed to persist over a period of years.

The problem of dandruff can be explained in exactly the same manner. If we are in full health, there is no excessive shedding of the dead cells. Conversely, such shedding is quite likely when a disease is present. In the overwhelming majority of cases, however, excessive shedding occurs even when no disease in full bloom is present. Here again it is the minor body imbalances, characteristic of living in the twilight zone of health, that are the most frequent causes of this condition.

Living in this gray zone has more serious and far-reaching consequences than merely the development of premature common baldness, premature common grayness, or dandruff. In the great majority of cases a full-blown disease does not strike suddenly. Minor body imbalances undermine resistance and may cause gradual deterioration of tissue, grooming the body, so to speak, for the development of a more serious malady. In the twilight zone of health the body is more susceptible to infectious diseases such as tuberculosis, influenza, and pneumonia. In addition, and much more important today, is the fact that living in the twilight zone of health may cause not only common baldness, common grayness, wrinkling, and other external characteristics of aging to develop sooner than need be, but also the premature degeneration of vital *internal* organs. This leads to such degenerative diseases as heart, circulatory and kidney diseases (arteriosclerosis), arthritis, diabetes, and possibly cancer. Degenerative diseases have all but defied medical science and are its major concern today, since infectious diseases can be avoided or cured for the most part through preventive vaccines and antibiotics.

Symptoms: Nature's Warnings

It has been pointed out that dandruff may develop and common baldness and common grayness may manifest themselves prematurely when we are in a state of disease or the twilight zone of health. At this point the question arises: how do we know when we are in either of these states?

When we are in full health, we are aware of it, because of the sense of well being we feel. Similarly, when we are in a state of something less than full health, we realize it through nature's warnings, or, as a doctor would say, from symptoms. A symptom may be defined as "a phenomenon which arises from and accompanies a particular disease or disorder and serves as an indication of it." Here is a list of common symptoms:

Headaches	Nervousness
Dizziness	Irritability
Heartburn	Twitching of eyelids or mouth
Gastric pain	
Abdominal pain	Muscular aches
Gall-bladder pain	Soreness of body joints
Gas	
Nausea	Breathlessness
Vomiting	Chest pain
Paleness	Dandruff
Abnormal loss of weight	Abnormal oiliness
	Abnormally dry scalp
Abnormal tiredness	Skin trouble
Sleeplessness	
Mental depression	

Note that dandruff, along with several other common maladies of the scalp, is listed. They are symptoms just as headaches or dizziness are symptoms, even though they may not cause any physical discomfort. Common baldness and common grayness could also be included in this list if they are developing prematurely, because their premature development is also a symptom of a body imbalance.

The presence of one or more of these symptoms is a sign of a body imbalance, serious or slight. It is not the occasional occurrence of any of these symptoms but their persistent presence about which we should be concerned.

Note, however, that some persons are born with or acquire unchangeable defects that result in chronic symptoms which must be recognized for what they are. A person born with an asthmatic condition, for example, may suffer from breathlessness. The symptom of breathlessness cannot be considered abnormal in this individual. *Each of us has a biologic normalcy at any point in time; it is this that we should try to maintain, for this is full health to us.*

Note also that, simply because most persons around us may be living in the twilight zone of health, it does not mean that this should be accepted as a normal consequence of living. It is possible to meet the challenges of life and still maintain full health.

CHAPTER 15

Baldness, Grayness, Dandruff --- Treatable or Nontreatable?

In an effort to answer the question whether baldness, grayness, and dandruff are treatable, we digressed occasionally along the way into seemingly unrelated areas. Each step was necessary, however, in order to present a complete picture in its proper perspective.

It is the purpose of this last chapter to correlate the important implications that have been presented and to spell out more specifically the only effective approach to common baldness, common grayness, dandruff, and healthy hair.

Baldness and Grayness

Are baldness and grayness treatable?

To answer this question we first had to learn that there are several types of these problems, some of which could be directly classified as treatable and others as nontreatable. Attention was focused on common baldness and common grayness because they could not be classified directly as either treatable or nontreatable and because they are the cause of most of the confusion and quackery that exists in the field of hair problems.

We pointed out that common baldness and common grayness are characteristics of aging which are fundamentally manifestations of the aging process, but it is heredity that largely determines when and how they will manifest themselves. They cannot be prevented from occurring, just as growing old cannot be prevented. We found, however, that they are treatable when they are developing prematurely.

The question that emerged at this point which had to be answered was: how can one determine whether or not common baldness and common grayness are in fact developing prematurely?

From the explanation in the previous chapter, we learned that only when we are in full health will these conditions not develop prematurely. If we are in a state of disease or in the twilight zone of health (which is characterized by minor body imbalances), these characteristics of aging may develop sooner than called for by our genetic makeup.

The next question that emerged was: how do we know when we are in the state of disease or in the twilight zone of health?

We pointed out that we become aware of being in a state of something less than full health through symptoms, which are nature's warnings of a body imbalance, serious or slight.

This completes the review of our findings about common baldness and common grayness. The situation resolves itself as follows:

1. If you are in full health (having no symptoms plaguing you), you must accept the development of common baldness and common grayness as natural manifestations of the aging process.

2. If you are in a state of disease which is undermining the body's resources, these characteristics of aging and others may be developing prematurely and, until the disease is cured and full health re-established, they may continue to do so.

3. If you are free from a full-blown disease but still not in a state of full health because there are one or more

symptoms plaguing you, then you are in the twilight zone of health, which is characterized by minor body imbalances. A minor body imbalance can undermine the body's resources and may cause common baldness and common grayness to develop prematurely, just as disease can. And, until the imbalance is eliminated, these characteristics of aging and others may continue to develop prematurely.

Dandruff

Is dandruff treatable?

In our coverage of scaliness, it was pointed out that there is common scurf, which is normal shedding of the epidermis, and there is dandruff, which is excessive shedding. Common scurf is fundamentally nontreatable. Dandruff is treatable because the excessive shedding is an abnormality which can be remedied. More specifically, dandruff was classified as a treatable symptomatic disorder because it is a symptom of a body imbalance, serious or slight, which can be remedied. Like other symptoms, dandruff often comes and goes. When it is not the symptom of a full-blown disease, it is a symptom caused by a minor body imbalance, characteristic of living in the twilight zone of health. Until the body imbalance is eliminated, the excessive shedding will persist.

Because it is within the twilight zone of health that most of us find ourselves, the discussion that follows spotlights some of the ramifications of living in this condition.

Between Health and Disease

The twilight zone of health was pointed out as being a condition in which we cannot be considered healthy within our potentiality nor can we be considered diseased by all practical standards.

We will probably never know at any point in time how many people are living in this gray zone. If you ever doubt, however, that the number runs into the millions, stop to consider the tons of symptomatic remedies being sold today on the American scene. Leading the list are aspirin tablets, upset stomach and constipation remedies, food supplements, vitamins, tonics, reducing aids, tranquilizers, and sleeping pills. If yours is the average household, the medicine cabinet is cluttered with such "remedies" and "aids."

While it is true that these products have worthwhile purposes, there is strong evidence that they are being used indiscriminately. Too many people allow the cause of their symptoms to go unquestioned, ignoring nature's warnings of a body imbalance which could be serious or could lead to a serious disease. Not only is their zest for living and productivity undermined, but they seem to be unaware that they may be permitting themselves to grow old before their time. Most people desire youthfulness and long life but seem to ignore the logical path which would lead them to the realization of these goals.

Such foolishness in treating body imbalances symptomatically will be illustrated in the following discussion on the relationship between symptoms and causes. If we learn to understand this simple relationship, we will have come to realize the only effective approach to premature common baldness, premature common grayness, dandruff, and healthy hair.

Symptoms and Causes

When the body is in a diseased state, there are always three factors present: (1) the underlying cause, (2) the body imbalance, and (3) the symptoms.

When a virus invades your system, for example, your temperature rises as your body mobilizes to counteract the infection. You become aware of this going on through symptoms, such as feeling hot and tired.

In this example, the underlying cause is the virus, the body imbalance is the rise in temperature (fever), and the symptoms are feeling hot and tired.

These three factors are always present whenever the body is affected by an adversity to which it cannot readily adapt.

In the case of a minor body imbalance (characteristic of living in the twilight zone of health), we find that the relationship is the same.

If you suffer from anxiety (emotional tension), for instance, your body may react by developing high blood pressure. You may become aware of this through symptoms such as headaches and tiredness.

In this example, the underlying cause is the anxiety, the body imbalance is the high blood pressure, and the symptoms are the headaches and tiredness.

Ordinarily, when you are in a state of disease or twilight zone of health, you are not aware of all three of these basic factors. You become aware of the symptoms readily but may not realize the nature of the body imbalance or its underlying cause. As in the preceding example, the symptoms of headaches and tiredness afflict you and are your immediate concern, but you may not realize that they were caused by the anxiety.

In any event, if you wish to eliminate the symptoms of headaches and tiredness, you must counteract the body imbalance, the high blood pressure. Obviously the only effective way of doing this is to remove the underlying cause, which is in this case the anxiety. Of course you can temporarily relieve the headaches with aspirin and the tiredness with rest, but the recurrence of the symptoms is inevitable, as long as the high blood pressure and the anxiety exist.

In the previous chapter three lists were included. List A itemized common underlying causes, List B common minor body imbalances, and List C some of the common symptoms.

The list of symptoms included dandruff along with several other hair problems, and, as indicated, would also include common baldness and common grayness when they are developing prematurely.

If you wish to eliminate any of these hair problems, as well as any other symptom, you must detect and counteract the causative body imbalance, such as those in List B. The only effective way of doing this would be to detect and remove the underlying cause, such as those in List A.

Of course you can temporarily wash away dandruff or resort to tints for grayness. Foolishly, though, you may try to cure baldness, grayness, or dandruff with "special" tonics and shampoos, or scalp treatments which may involve the use of ultraviolet light, high-frequency stimulation, vibration apparatus, suction cups, "secret" ointments and lotions, "special" massaging and plucking techniques, and so on. However, the premature development of common baldness or common grayness, or the excessive shedding of dandruff will persist, as long as the body imbalance and its underlying cause exist.

Similarly, ordinary brushing, massaging, and shampooing will not cure baldness, grayness or dandruff, although they help keep the hair and scalp well groomed and aid in providing a healthy environment for normal hair growth.

Any ailment, serious or slight, should fall within the sphere of the physician. Any special symptomatic scalp treatment, therefore, should always be administered under direct medical supervision. *But even medically supervised symptomatic treatment without removing the underlying cause will be in vain.*

Mere symptomatic treatment is similar to foolishly patching a leaking ceiling as water continues to overflow from a stopped sink on the floor above. Just as we must remove the underlying cause to eliminate a body imbalance and its symptoms, we must first unstop the sink to eliminate the overflowing water and leaking ceiling.

In Retrospect

Having captured the essence of what has been written here, you have joined the ranks of the few who know the answers to the questions about hair problems which have baffled curious men and women for centuries.

When thoroughly dissected and recognized for what they are, the problems of common baldness, common grayness, and dandruff are not as inexplicable as heretofore considered.

Unfortunately, the uninformed continue to yield to superstition and quackery and remain unaware of the important significance of these problems—that is, their relationship to aging and the state of health.

All of us must realize that, contrary to claims by some in the worlds of business and science, health and beauty are not purchasable, and that instead, we must correct the mismanagements of our everyday life or other remediable causes which keep us in the twilight zone of health and lead not only to premature common baldness, premature common grayness, dandruff and the like, but also to degenerative diseases, a much more serious scourge to modern man.